Personalized Cancer Chemotherapy

Personalized Cancer Chemotherapy

An Effective Way of Enhancing Outcomes in Clinics

Da-Yong Lu

ELSEVIER

AMSTERDAM • BOSTON • CAMBRIDGE • HEIDELBERG
LONDON • NEW YORK • OXFORD • PARIS • SAN DIEGO
SAN FRANCISCO • SINGAPORE • SYDNEY • TOKYO
Woodhead Publishing is an imprint of Elsevier

WP
WOODHEAD
PUBLISHING

Woodhead Publishing is an imprint of Elsevier
80 High Street, Sawston, Cambridge, CB22 3HJ, UK
225 Wyman Street, Waltham, MA 02451, USA
Langford Lane, Kidlington, OX5 1GB, UK

British Library Cataloguing in Publication Data
A catalogue record for this book is available from the British Library

Library of Congress Control Number: 2014957608

ISBN: 978-0-08-100346-6

For information on all Woodhead Publishing publications visit our website at http://store.elsevier.com/

Typeset by TNQ Books and Journals
www.tnq.co.in

Contents

List of figures and tables

Figures

Tables

About the author

Dr Da-Yong Lu, born July 1962 Shanghai. Associate professor.

Ed PhD, Shanghai Institute of Materia Medica, Chinese Academy of Sciences, 2005; MS, Shanghai Institute of Materia Medica, Chinese Academy of Sciences, 1986; BS, Shanghai Medical University (now Fudan University) 1982. Currently associated professor at Shanghai University, China. He has studied cancer pathology, biochemistry, pharmacology and clinical therapeutics, especially the pharmacological studies of new Chinese anticancer agents probimane and MST-16, antimetastatic targeting of fibrinogen and sialic acids and individualized cancer chemotherapy (ICC), since 1982 and some articles on avian flu, AIDS and neural science. His interest is focused on basic studies of cancer biology, pathology and treatment, origins of life and some other fields. He is an editor for several reputed international journals. More than 50 of his original articles have been published in international journals.

Professor and Dr Da-Yong Lu, Shanghai University, Shanghai 200444, PR China
email: ludayong@sh163.net or ludayong@shu.edu.cn

Preface

When I was a college student in Shanghai Medical University in 1980, I dreamed of finding a new drug to banish all cancers. However, when I went to the Shanghai Institute of Materia Medica, Chinese Academy of Sciences, for graduate study of anticancer drug pharmacology in 1982, I began to realize that cancers are different diseases that need treating with different drugs. Furthermore, we often do not know which anticancer drug is the best one when we face a specific cancer patient in a clinic. So I began my journey in individualized cancer chemotherapy in the following years, most intensively since 2005. Now, after more than 30 years of focus on this topic, I offer this book to bring the problem to readers, who I hope can benefit and advance their knowledge of ICC.

Clinical cancer chemotherapy is unsatisfactory and far from perfect. Many cancer patients die still, in spite of it. One of the major obstacles to controlling cancer growth and metastases in patients is the inappropriate use of anticancer and antimetastatic drugs. As increasing numbers and types of anticancer drugs are developed, clinicians become more and more likely to misuse anticancer or antimetastatic drugs in their practice. The present norm is to use a chemotherapeutic regimen that is 'randomized' or 'standard' in relation to the target organ or tumor origin. Since cancers can originate from a wide variety of genetically or phenotypically abnormal genes, molecules and tissues, they ought to be sensitive to different anticancer drugs. Thus, most cancer patients are unsuited to the use of such 'uniform' or 'standardized' chemotherapy. As no single drug or drug combination has so far been found to be optimal for cancers of all origins, developing a good and clinically practical drug selection system is no less important than the discovery and development of new anticancer drugs. Researchers and clinicians are now beginning to focus on 'individualized cancer chemotherapy' (ICC) also called 'personalized cancer chemotherapy' (PCC), with the intention of improving therapeutic quality and outcomes by selecting and prescribing the best matched drugs (the 'right' anticancer drugs) and avoiding ineffective anticancer drugs. Given a knowledge of relationships between drug responses and the genetic pathogenic status of a specific tumor, physicians can prescribe the possibly best-matched anticancer drugs in succeeding trials. Present understandings of the relationship between drug response and tumor growth or metastases are not well-established, but there are generally two ways of extracting information on these relationships from tumors in clinics:

1. drug sensitivity testing;
2. tumor genetic, molecular or bioinformatics, from obtained tumor tissues.

The first experiments relating to this issue date back to the early 1950s [1,2]. Those reports provided the experimental basis for evaluating drug sensitivity in tumor samples from humans. Systematic investigations of drug sensitivity tests in clinics began in the late 1970s [3–5]. Since then, drug sensitivity tests have been the mainstream of ICC strategy and continue to be one of the best-known resources for modifying selection of chemotherapeutic agents in current clinical practice. However, much clinical practice in respect of drug sensitivity testing is unsatisfactory, especially regarding survival rates in late stage cancer patients. The gradual transformation from drug sensitivity testing to cancer biomarker detection and pharmacogenetics is a contemporary and future trend.

At the start of the 21st century, the genetic abnormalities related to cancer etiology and therapeutics have become easier to identify and detect accurately [6–8], and there has been a new trend towards utilizing these cancer biomarkers and bioinformatics data as selective criteria for predicting drug responses [6–12]. Benefiting from the Human Genome Project (HGP) and post-HGP, the use of these techniques is growing rapidly [13]. Using genetic, molecular and bioinformatics data and modern experimental techniques, known tumor genes can be detected more easily than ever before; the average speed of genetic sequencing has increased 15,000 to 50,000 times over the time of HGP ten years ago. These techniques will be used in ICC strategies far and wide and in future clinical utilizations [13–15].

Pharmacogenetics also addresses which drug might work in an individual patient, and at what dosage; and if a given type of anticancer drug is suitable for a specific individual or tumors [16–19]. These types of research can meet some of the requirements of individualized therapy. This type of study is presently the major ICC strategy. It will soon be, however, unlikely to be used alone to reach a well-received therapeutic outcome. Further information and reasons are given in the following sections.

The major misconception of work in individualized cancer chemotherapy today is that it is mostly designed to receive information on and target primary tumors. However, 90% of cancer patients die of metastasis. So although primary tumors are being inhibited by antiproliferative or cytotoxic anticancer drugs, patients' survival rates have been increased very little. In order to improve this situation, we shall shift focus to the development of effective antimetastatic drugs and individualized cancer chemotherapy on patients' metastases as a future trend, especially for some late-stage cancer patients [20–23]. In this book, we delineate different strategies of individualized antimetastatic therapy and emphasize it with new twists.

Most cancers have multiple genetic alterations or abnormalities [24,25]. Using only one anticancer drug in clinical cancer cases is seldom very useful. Anticancer drug combination is better than a single drug in most situations [26–28]. How to combine anticancer drugs is a new area of anticancer drug therapy. Presumably, the best strategy is an anticancer drug treatment cocktail, such as the use of highly cytotoxic chemicals with biotherapies [28]. If highly cytotoxic chemicals can easily kill 70% to 90% of tumor cells, the highly specific biotherapies will be designed to kill the rest [8,28]. On the other hand, combining the utilization of antiproliferative drugs with antimetastatic drugs is also promising. It is expected that strategies of these kinds will be good paradigms for future cancer chemotherapy.

The causes for the death of cancer patients treated in clinics can be multi-factorial. Apart from direct causes from tumor progression, other clinical complications or psychiatric factors will hasten the deaths of cancer patients to a greater or lesser extent. So many assistant therapies will be administered to the patients who have some clinical complications, blood coagulation status [29,30] or psychiatric problems or physical weakness. There are many success stories about the use of such therapies in clinics in enhancing patients' survival rates.

Cost-effectiveness is a long-standing medical issue and is also an early concern of mathematics in ICC. Increasing efforts to develop ICC are generally paralleled by rising diagnostic costs. Systematic evaluation of the relationship between the running costs and benefits of ICC is crucial for updating the ICC system and making it available in the long run, since the cost of therapy is a critical matter. The balance between cost and effectiveness is an unavoidable part of any ICC research project and cannot be overlooked. The consideration of how to increase good therapeutic outcomes with limited funds is an important task for cancer chemotherapy development.

It has been six decades since the first individualized cancer chemotherapy was introduced. More and more individualized cancer chemotherapy strategies have been devised and systematically researched. Since we cannot possibly use all of these strategies in one patient, we must decide which ICC strategy is the best. Each has its own advantages and disadvantages. At present, the major obstacles of cancer chemotherapy are the development of drug resistance, severe side effects and tumor metastasis. Owing to the modest tumor specificity of many anticancer drugs, normal tissues are also damaged. This prevents the application of sufficiently high doses to eradicate less sensitive tumor-cell populations or clones. Thereby, tumors develop drug resistance, leading to treatment failure and fatal consequences. Cancer metastasis, as noted, is responsible for 90% of cancer deaths. So in this book, a chapter is devoted to individualized antimetastatic strategies and drug combinations. The development of more research in this area will be invaluable for cancer therapy.

Although different strategies of ICC have been designed according to different technological systems, no available strategy has been generally effective enough to significantly increase patients' survival compared with conventional therapy, possibly owing to chemotherapy's targeting of primary rather than metastatic tumors. So we desperately need to streamline present ICC strategies and create new types of ICC strategies, then to integrate the advantages of all ICC types, especially in designing systems to predict drug response to formed metastatic nodules [31]. Although great efforts have been made in fulfilling ICC, many significant obstacles still remain to be surmounted. Are we ready yet to perfect a balanced and effective, life-saving strategy? [32]

In this book, we separately describe and address these ICC strategies new and old, to provide readers with new insight. Your feedback will be welcomed, so that we can progress towards perfecting these ICC strategies and hopefully saving the lives of more cancer patients.

References

[1] M.M. Black, F.D. Speer, Further observations on the effects of cancer chemotherapeutic agents on the in vitro dehydrogenase activity of cancer tissue, J. Natl. Cancer Inst. 14 (5) (1954) 1147–58.
[2] J.C. Wright, J.P. Cobb, S.L. Gumport, F.M. Golomb, D. Safadi, Investigation of the relation between clinical and tissue-Culture response to chemotherapeutic agents on human cancer, N. Eng. J. Med. 257 (25) (1957) 1207–11.
[3] A.W. Hamburger, S.E. Salmon, Primary bioassay of human tumor stem cells, Science (Washington DC) 197 (4302) (1977) 461–3.
[4] S.E. Salmon, A.W. Hamburger, B. Soehnlen, B.G.M. Durie, D.S. Alberts, T.E. Moon, Quantitation of differential sensitivity of human-tumor stem cells to anticancer drugs, N. Eng. J. Med. 298 (1978) 1321–7.
[5] A. Bogden, A rapid screening method for testing chemotherapeutic agents against human tumour xenografts, in: D.O.A. Houchens (Ed.), Proceedings of the Symposium of the Use of Athymic (Nude) Mice in Cancer Research, Gustav Fischer Inc, New York, 1978, pp. 231–50.
[6] R.L. Strausberg, A.J.G. Simpson, L.J. Old, G.J. Riggins, Oncogenomics and the development of new cancer therapies, Nature 429 (2004) 469–74.
[7] D.Y. Lu, X. L. Chen, J. Ding, Individualized cancer chemotherapy integrating drug sensitivity tests, pathological profile analysis and computational coordination-an effective strategy to improve clinical treatment, Med. Hypotheses 66 (1) (2006) 45–51.
[8] D.Y. Lu, T.R. Lu, X.L. Chen, J. Ding, Individualized Cancer chemotherapy, in: M.M. Shoja, P.S. Agutter, R.S. Tubbs, M. Ghanei, K. Ghabili et al. (Eds.), Hypotheses in Clinical Medicine, Chapter 13, Nova science publishers, Hauppage, NY, 2012.
[9] W.S. Dalton, S.H. Friend, Cancer biomarkers – an invitation to the Table, Science 312 (5777) (2006) 1165–8.
[10] A. Ocana, A. Pandiella, Personalized therapies in the cancer "omics" era, Mol. Cancer 9 (2010) 202.
[11] B. Stransky, P. Galante, Application of bioinformatics in cancer research, in: W.C.S. Cho (Ed.), An OMICS Perspective on Cancer Research. 12, Springer, Dordrecht, NL, 2010, pp. 211–33.
[12] D.Y. Lu, T.R. Lu, S. Cao, Individualized cancer chemotherapy by detecting cancer biomarkers, Metabolomics 2 (5) (2012) e121.
[13] E.S. Lander, Initial impact of the sequencing of the human genome, Nature 470 (2011) 187–97.
[14] F. Collins, Has the revolution arrived? Nature 464 (2010) 674–5.
[15] J.C. Venter, Multiple personal genomes await, Nature 464 (2010) 676–7.
[16] J.W. Watters, H.L. McLeod, Cancer pharmacogenomics: current and future applications, Biochim. Biophys. Acta 1603 (2) (2003) 99–111.
[17] T. Efferth, M. Volm, Pharmacogenetics for individualized cancer chemotherapy, Pharmacol. Ther. 107 (2) (2005) 155–76.
[18] J.F. Deeken, W.D. Figg, S.E. Bates, A. Sparreboom, Toward individualized treatment: prediction of anticancer drug disposition and toxicity with pharmacogenetics, Anticancer Drugs 18 (2) (2007) 111–26.
[19] R.S. Huang, M. J Ratain, Pharmacogenetics and pharmacogenomics of anticancer agents, CA Cancer J. Clin. 59 (1) (2009) 42–55.
[20] G.P. Gupta, J. Massagué, Cancer metastasis: building a framework, Cell 127 (2006) 679–95.

[21] S. Valastyan, R.A. Weinberg, Tumor metastasis: molecular insights and evolving paradigms, Cell 147 (2) (2011) 275–92.
[22] D.Y. Lu, T.R. Lu, S. Cao, Cancer metastases and clinical therapies, Cell Dev. Biol. 1 (4) (2012) e110.
[23] D.Y. Lu, T.R. Lu, H.Y. Wu, New insights into individualized antimetastatic therapy, Adv. Tech. Biol. Med. 1 (1) (2013) 106.
[24] P.C. Nowell, The clonal evolution of tumor cell populations, Science (Washington DC) 194 (4260) (1976) 23–8.
[25] D. Hanahan, R.A. Weinberg, The hallmarks of cancer, Cell 100 (1) (2000) 57–70.
[26] A.J. Tipping, J.V. Melo, Imatinib mesylate in combination with other chemotherapeutic drugs: in vitro studies, Semin. Hematol. 40 (2 Suppl 2) (2003) 83–91.
[27] B.J. Druker, Imatinib alone and in combination for chronic myeloid leukemia, Semin. Hematol. 40 (1) (2003) 50–8.
[28] D.Y. Lu, T.R. Lu, H. Y. Wu, Combination chemical agents with biological means in cancer therapy, Researches Rev. BioSci. 7 (4) (2013) 153–5.
[29] M. Mandala, G. Ferretti, M. Cremonesi, M. Cazzaniga, G. Curigliano, S. Barni, Venous thromboembolism and cancer: new issues for an old topic, Crit. Rev. Oncol. Hematol. 48 (1) (2003) 65–80.
[30] D.Y. Lu, X. L. Chen, J. Ding, Treatment of solid tumors and metastases by fibrinogen-targeted anticancer drug therapy, Med. Hypotheses. 68 (1) (2007) 188–93.
[31] D.Y. Lu, T.R. Lu, H.Y. Wu, S. Cao, Cancer metastases treatment, Curr. Drug. Ther. 8 (1) (2013) 24–9.
[32] D.Y. Lu, T.R. Lu, X.L. Chen, Individualized Cancer chemotherapy, are We ready for that yet? Metabolomics 2 (2012) e113.

List of abbreviations

Bcl	B-cell lymphoma
CAM	complementary and alternative medicine
CYP	cytochrome P-450
EGF	epidermal growth factor
EMT	epithelial-mesenchymal transition
HER2	human epidermal growth factor
HIF	hypoxia-inducible factors
ICER	incremental cost-effectiveness ratio
LMWH	low molecular weight heparin
MDR	multidrug resistance
MET	mesenchymal-epithelial transition
MMP	matrix metalloproteinase
QALY	quality-adjusted life-years
SNP	single nucleotide polymorphism
TCM	Traditional Chinese medicine
TNF	tumor necrosis factor
VEGF	vascular endothelial growth factor

Introduction

1

Cancer treatment is an unsolved, thorny problem. Cancer is one of the leading causes of human deaths all over the world. Paradoxically, given our expectations, we have achieved very little in this respect, despite the huge amount of money and human resources that have been expended. There is a plethora of reasons for this situation. Two are particularly important:

1. different cancers respond to different anticancer drugs and we cannot accurately predict responses to a given type of anticancer drug;
2. there is up to now no good way of treating tumor metastasis in clinics, especially on formed metastatic nodules.

To solve these two problems, we address, review and discuss many ideas for individualized cancer chemotherapy in clinics in this book with the hope that readers will have in-depth perspectives for these two problems, so as to be ready to find better answers to these and new challenges.

Cancer is a number of different diseases, all with the pathological feature of unlimited growth. The hallmarks of cancer can be many different genes and many different series of stages [1–2]. Since tumors originate from a widely varying background of genotypically or phenotypically abnormal tissues that cause the unlimited growth of cells, different genotypically or phenotypically abnormal tissues ought to be sensitive to and so matched with different anticancer drugs. Thus, most cancer patients are unsuited to the use of 'uniform' or 'standardized' chemotherapy [3–4]. As no single drug or combination has so far been found to be optimal for cancers of all origins, developing a good and clinically sensitive anticancer drug selection system is no less important than the discovery of new anticancer drugs. 'Individualized cancer chemotherapy' (ICC) or 'personal cancer chemotherapy' (PCC) is designed and tailored to meet this requirement of improving therapeutic quality by selecting and prescribing well-matched anticancer drugs and avoiding ineffective anticancer drugs by adopting a series of systematic methodologies in clinics [3–4].

The first experiments relating to this issue date back to the early 1950s [5–6]. Those reports hypothesized and testified the experimental basis for evaluating anticancer drug sensitivity to tumor samples obtained from human cancer tissue and offering the most sensitive anticancer drugs to these cancer patients—drug sensitivity testing. Systematic investigations and utilization of drug sensitivity tests in clinics began in the late 1970s [7–9]. Since then, drug sensitivity tests have been the mainstream of ICC strategy up to 2000, and continue to be one of the best means of selecting chemotherapeutic agents for future clinical practice. (Chapter 2)

Cancer is a disease of genetic alteration and abnormalities. The best therapeutic approaches should target these genetic alterations and abnormalities. However,

Personalized Cancer Chemotherapy.

different cancers are caused by different genetic alterations and abnormalities. Thus, before an appropriate therapy can be initiated, the exact genetic alterations and abnormalities of a specific cancer must be known in the treatment clinic. Only genetic, RNA or protein detection of these genetic alterations or abnormalities in tumor cells can offer the useful prediction of possible anticancer drug responses we need for individualized cancer chemotherapy. Genetic, RNA or protein detection of cancer represent the exact sites of oncogenic or metastatic processes and underpin modern individualized cancer chemotherapy. They can be divided into two general categories:

1. Detection of the quantities of tumor biomarkers at subquantitative or quantitative level to predict the use of anticancer drugs targeting the detection of increasing levels of oncogenic and metastatic molecules. We categorize this as 'detection of cancer biomarkers';
2. Detection of polymorphism of human or tumor genes to predict the anticancer drugs which will be active to tumor tissues and in human bodies. We categorize it as 'pharmacogenomics of anticancer drugs'.

In this book, two chapters (3 and 4) address these topics, including many basic rules relating to genetic, RNA, protein or glycol-protein detection for drug choice from detected oncogenic or metastatic sites in tumors and pharmacogenetics to predict drug doses, toxicity and responses to cancers.

Previously, cancer biomarker detections have been focused on one or several molecules (commonly protein or glycoprotein biomarkers such as HER-2) of tumor tissues in one patient. At the start of the 21st century, the genetic disorders related to cancer etiology and therapeutics have become easier to identify and detect in high throughput ways—cancer bioinformatics [3–4,10–14], and there has been a new trend towards utilizing these high throughput bioinformatics data as drug-selective criteria for ICC [3–4,10–14]. Using bioinformatics data and modern experimental techniques, known tumor gene or protein abnormality can be detected more easily and with higher throughput than ever before. The detected genetic molecules can be determined, at the highest, at as many as 70 genetic alleles in one test [13]. These types of techniques will be used widely in future. (Chapter 3)

Pharmacogenetics also predicts which drug might work in an individual patient, and at what dosage range, and if one type of anticancer drug is suitable for a specific cancer patient to have the drug metabolite in active concentrations [15–18]. These types of research can meet some of the requirements of selecting drugs that are potentially sensitive to an individual, but it is better to use this type of method with other ICC methods, such as drug sensitivity tests or tumor biomarker detections.

90% of cancer patients die of cancer metastasis. Currently, however, cancer chemotherapies are mainly focusing on anticancer drugs targeting the primary tumor, not the metastatic foci. So although primary tumors have been inhibited by sensitive antiproliferative drugs, patients' survival rates have been increased very little [4]. If we change our focus to the development of effective antimetastatic drugs and individualized cancer metastasis, chemotherapy strategies can be targeted for patients in late stages of cancer. Thus we might expect in future to enhance patients' survival rates with the use of individualized antimetastatic therapies [19–22]. Chapter 5.

Most cancers have multiple genetic alterations or abnormalities [1–2]. It is seldom very useful to use only one anticancer drug in clinical cancer treatment. Presumably, one of the best strategies is the combinatory use of anticancer drugs, especially combinations of chemicals and biotherapies or combinations of antiproliferative anticancer drugs with antimetastatic agents. If chemical anticancer drugs kill 70% to 90% of tumor cells, the highly specific biotherapies or antimetastatic drugs can kill the rest. It is expected that these strategies will be a paradigm in future cancer chemotherapy [4,23]. Chapter 6.

The causes of death of cancer patients can be multi-factorial in clinics. Apart from direct causes, from tumor progressions, other clinical complications (such as venous thrombosis) or psychiatric factors will speed the death of many cancer patients. So many assistant therapies have been developed, which help the patients who have some clinical complications or psychiatric issues [4] and considerably increase patients' survival rates. Chapter 7.

Cost-effectiveness is a long-standing medical problem and is also an early concern of mathematics in ICC. Increasing efforts to develop ICC are generally paralleled by rising diagnostic costs. Systematic evaluation of the relationship between the running costs and benefits of ICC is crucial in updating the ICC system and making it available in the long run, since the cost of therapy is a critical matter for patients and doctors to consider. From previous studies, many diagnostic methods can be shown as cost-effective, because the cost of cancer biomarker detection or gene polymorphism detection is commonly smaller than that of many anticancer drugs, or of time in hospital. If we use the right anticancer drugs, because we know the cancer biomarkers, patients' survival rates will increase substantially, especially in early stages [24]. Chapter 8.

Further information will be outlined in detail, discussed and concluded in the following sections. Chapters 9 and 10.

References

[1] P.C. Nowell, The clonal evolution of tumor cell populations, Science 194 (4260) (1976) 23–28 (Washington DC).

[2] D. Hanahan, R.A. Weinberg, The hallmarks of cancer, Cell 100 (1) (2000) 57–70.

[3] D.Y. Lu, X.L. Chen, J. Ding, Individualized cancer chemotherapy integrating drug sensitivity tests, pathological profile analysis and computational coordination-an effective strategy to improve clinical treatment, Med. Hypotheses 66 (1) (2006) 45–51.

[4] D.Y. Lu, T.R. Lu, X.L. Chen, J. Ding, Individualized Cancer Chemotherapy, in: M.M. Shoja, P.S. Agutter, R.S. Tubbs, M. Ghanei, K. Ghabili et al. (Eds.), Hypotheses in Clinical Medicine, Nova Science Publishers, Hauppage, NY, 2012. chapter 13.

[5] M.M. Black, F.D. Speer, Further observations on the effects of cancer chemotherapeutic agents on the in vitro dehydrogenase activity of cancer tissue, J. Natl. Cancer Inst. 14 (5) (1954) 1147–1158.

[6] J.C. Wright, J.P. Cobb, S.L. Gumport, F.M. Golomb, D. Safadi, Investigation of the relation between clinical and tissue-culture response to chemotherapeutic agents on human cancer, N. Eng. J. Med. 257 (25) (1957) 1207–1211.

[7] A.W. Hamburger, S.E. Salmon, Primary bioassay of human tumor stem cells, Science 197 (1977) 461–463 (Washington DC).
[8] S.E. Salmon, A.W. Hamburger, B. Soehnlen, B.G.M. Durie, D.S. Alberts, T.E. Moon, Quantitation of differential sensitivity of human-tumor stem cells to anticancer drugs, N. Eng. J. Med. 298 (1978) 1321–1327.
[9] A. Bogden, A rapid screening method for testing chemotherapeutic agents against human tumour xenografts, in: D.O.A. Houchens (Ed.), Proceedings of the Symposium of the use of Athymic (Nude) Mice in Cancer Research, Gustav Fischer Inc, New York, 1978, pp. 231–250.
[10] W.S. Dalton, S.H. Friend, Cancer biomarkers – an invitation to the table, Science 312 (5777) (2006) 1165–1168.
[11] A. Ocana, A. Pandiella, Personalized therapies in the cancer "omics" era, Mol. Cancer 9 (2010) 202.
[12] B. Stransky, P. Galante, Application of Bioinformatics in Cancer Research, in: W.C.S. Cho (Ed.), An OMICS Perspective on Cancer Research, 12, Springer, Dordrecht, NL, 2010, pp. 211–233.
[13] V.P. Retèl, M.A. Joore, M. Knauer, S.C. Linn, M. Hauptmann, et al., Cost-effectiveness of the 70-gene signature versus St. Gallen guidelines and adjuvant online for early breast cancer, European J. Cancer 46 (8) (2010) 1382–1391.
[14] D.Y. Lu, T.R. Lu, S. Cao, Individualized cancer chemotherapy by detecting cancer biomarkers, Metabolomics 2 (5) (2012) e121.
[15] J.W. Watters, H.L. McLeod, Cancer pharmacogenomics: current and future applications, Biochim. Biophys. Acta 1603 (2) (2003) 99–111.
[16] T. Efferth, M. Volm, Pharmacogenetics for individualized cancer chemotherapy, Pharmacol. Ther. 107 (2) (2005) 155–176.
[17] J.F. Deeken, W.D. Figg, S.E. Bates, A. Sparreboom, Toward individualized treatment: prediction of anticancer drug disposition and toxicity with pharmacogenetics, Anticancer Drugs 18 (2) (2007) 111–126.
[18] R.S. Huang, M.J. Ratain, Pharmacogenetics and pharmacogenomics of anticancer agents, CA: A Cancer J. Clin. 59 (1) (2009) 42–55.
[19] D.Y. Lu, T.R. Lu, S. Cao, Cancer metastases and clinical therapies, Cell & Dev. Bio. 1 (4) (2012) e110.
[20] S. Valastyan, R.A. Weinberg, Tumor metastasis: Molecular insights and evolving paradigms, Cell 147 (2) (2011) 275–292.
[21] D.Y. Lu, T.R. Lu, H.Y. Wu, New insights into individualized antimetastatic therapy, Adv. Tech. Biol. Med. 1 (1) (2013) 106.
[22] D.Y. Lu, T.R. Lu, H.Y. Wu, S. Cao, Cancer metastases treatment, Current Drug Therapy 8 (1) (2013) 24–29.
[23] D.Y. Lu, T.R. Lu, H.Y. Wu, Combination chemical agents with biological means in cancer therapy, Researches and Reviews in BioScience 7 (4) (2013) 153–155.
[24] A. Naeim, E.B. Keeler, Is adjuvant therapy for older patients with node (-) early breast cancer cost-effective? Crit. Rev. Oncol. Hematol. 53 (1) (2005) 81–89.

Drug sensitivity testing

2

2.1 History of drug sensitivity testing

Individualized cancer chemotherapy (ICC) was pioneered in drug sensitivity tests more than half a century ago [1–2]. It garnered more attention and received a boost during the 1970s [3–5]. In a drug sensitivity test the anticancer actions of candidate drugs on surgically removed tumor samples are compared, and the drugs showing the best responses are selected for use in succeeding treatments. Individualized cancer chemotherapy deployed before 2000 is generally regarded as drug sensitivity testing. Although anticancer drug sensitivity testing (DST) is the forerunner of ICC, its beneficial to clinical cancer patients is presently controversial. Despite DST techniques are diversified, innovated and improved a great deal in the past several decade, they are not developed into powerful means to cure all cancer patients. Much effort is needed for updating DST technology and hospital routines in future.

2.2 Methodology of drug sensitivity testing [6–7]

Drug sensitivity tests can be conducted *in vivo* and *in vitro*. The subrenal capsule (SRC) assay [5] is the earliest and best known *in vivo* method. It involves transplanting surgically removed tumors into the renal capsules of mice and evaluating the candidate anticancer drugs within 4-11 days. *In vitro* drug sensitivity testing methods involve cytological or cyto-chemical evaluations of drug response tests and include the micro-culture tetrazolium (MTT) method [8–9] , the ChemoFx method [10], the ATP luminescence assay [11–13], the collagen gel droplet-embedded culture method [14] and many others. Usually, the effects of drugs on tumor enzyme activity, energy consumption or cell numbers are assessed for different *in vitro* drug sensitivity testing. For example, Kondo and colleagues described a test involving drug effects on succinate dehydrogenase activity in tumors [15]; this was the prototype of the currently used MTT method. To reduce interference by normal cells collected along with the neoplastic tissue, serum-free culture is recommended to promote and test tumor growth selectively [11].

Theoretically, all *in vitro* drug sensitivity test methods exhibit similar biological or pharmacological features (inhibition of tumor cell proliferation). Their differences are the subtly different environmental conditions that tumor cells live in. These differences in environmental condition do not alter the core of a drug sensitivity test. So overall, these drug sensitivity tests should all be useable and drug response rates ought not to vary greatly in clinical chemotherapy.

The success or failure of a chemotherapy regime is determined by a number of clonal or stem cells in tumor tissue [16]. Thus drug sensitivity tests aimed at determining drug

Personalized Cancer Chemotherapy.

response in clonal or stem cells might be more useful or correct for predicting drug response in a tumor tissue. In future, a new stage of *in vitro* drug sensitivity testing should prioritize these tumor cell types to be more accurate and hence more effective.

2.3 Comparison between *in vivo* and *in vitro* drug sensitivity testing methodologies [6–7]

The major perceived advantage of the SRC assay is based on the assumption that the drug sensitivity testing is conducted on a tumor within a living body. The environment of the renal capsule has been proposed as more relevant to clinical situations than *in vitro* drug sensitivity tests. *In vitro* drug sensitivity testing lacks the activation or inactivation of human liver enzymes. Although some rat hepatic metabolizing enzymes (rat liver homogenizers) are used to activate or inactivate anticancer drugs, anticancer drug metabolism in cancer patients is still different. This method was once widely practiced and studied but its use has declined. Its disadvantages are as follows:

1. It is labor-intensive and technically demanding. A routine SRC assay needs three skilled personnel working for 2 to 4 hours. The high cost of hiring skilled personnel makes it cannot easily be widely used. As well as this, a sufficiently pathogen-free laboratory space for breeding immune-deficient nude mice on a large scale, as well as other operational spaces, are seldom available in conventional hospitals. Therefore, only small numbers of nude mice can be provided and very limited numbers of patients can be tested by this method.
2. Limits on the numbers of drugs usable for drug sensitivity or response tests make it difficult to select well-matched drugs from the limited candidate anticancer drug panel. The maximum number of drugs tested in one screening for SRC assay is 4 to 6, and it seems unlikely that the best-suited anticancer drugs will be among those 4 to 6 anticancer drugs. The likelihood of selecting the 'best' options is less than optimal.
3. The SRC assay does not always improve chemotherapy outcomes compared to *in vitro* drug sensitivity testing, especially in clinical practice for patients' survival [16]. The other main disadvantage is the financial burden of the SRC assay, in terms of the clinical use of immunodeficient nude mice and the hiring of specialized personnel [7].

Previously, several attempts to supersede the utilization of costly nude mice with that of relatively low-priced normal mice have been proposed [17–19]. There has been a longstanding controversy over whether athymic nude mice differ from immunocompetent normal mice in drug sensitivity tests. It was found that xenografts of primary surgical explants showed more positive tumor growth rate and drug response rate in 4 to 6 days in immunocompetent mice (82%) than in an 11-day SRC assay in nude mice (30%) [18–19]. We have suggested that drug response rates in normal and nude mice are the same if the experiment is terminated in the same period of time (4 to 7 days) [20]. It is likely that the differences between SRC assay results are more closely related to the duration of the experiment than to the immunological status of the tumor recipient. However, the duration should be no longer than seven days in immunocompetent mice as immune rejection may ensue.

The advantage of many *in vitro* drug sensitivity tests is that they are easier to perform and can be implemented in a routine hospital, so it is much less difficult to use them in daily hospital routine and practice. For these reasons, they are now the preferred method. The disadvantage of standard *in vitro* drug sensitivity tests is that they lack a matrix and other environmental resources to support solid tumor growth and do not deliver information on the metabolism of anticancer drugs in human bodies. However, most patients undergoing chemotherapy in clinics carry solid tumors, which are different from the material used in *in vitro* drug sensitivity testing situations. Some types of anticancer drugs, especially antimetastatic drugs targeting aspects of the tumor matrix and environment, such as the fibrinogen-related pathway, will elicit little or no response in *in vitro* drug sensitivity systems. More recently, some types of *in vitro* drug sensitivity tests have been supplemented with a tumor matrix in culture [14]. With further scientific and technological developments, new types of *in vitro* drug sensitivity tests will meet clinical requirements more perfectly and will be used to test drug responses in environments resembling natural ones. Overall, the drug responses in *in vivo* and *in vitro* drug sensitivity are theoretically the same. The new state-of-the-art *in vitro* drug sensitivity testing might be more suitable for clinical applications.

2.4 Relationship of drug responses in drug chemosensitivity testing and clinical tumor treatment

In approximately 80% of clinical reports solid relationships are shown between the results of drug sensitivity testing and clinical drug responses (PR or CR). Most clinical data show that drug responses in drug sensitivity testing are parallel with drug responses in cancer patients in clinics. In most cases, drug responses (PR or CR) in cancer patients are improved in comparison with the results of drug sensitivity testing. However, only 25-35% of clinical reports at most showed improvements in patients' survival through the use of drug sensitivity tests. In most cases, survival rates are almost the same whether drug sensitivity testing is used or not [7].

2.5 Possible reasons for unsatisfactory survival rates in spite of using drug sensitivity testing

The following three reasons can be postulated for unsatisfactory survival rates in spite of using *in vivo* or *in vitro* drug sensitivity testing:

(i) inappropriate use of the methodology and techniques of drug sensitivity testing
(ii) tumor tissues easily acquire multidrug resistance (MDR), and then regrow after a short period of inhibition and patients die normally
(iii) chemotherapy is not targeted on neoplasm metastases.

2.5.1 Technical analysis of protocols of drug sensitivity testing

Many factors, including technical details, determine the success or failure of a drug sensitivity test. Any neglect of experimental details will lead to complete failure of the test. The purpose of these tests is the accurate selection of anticancer drugs. Previously, many reports compared the sensitivity of 2 to 5 anticancer drugs, using only one dosage (concentration). The most suitable drug, however, may not be among these 2 to 5 anticancer drugs, nor may the correct dose be in the range used in a drug sensitivity test. It might be impossible to select the best drugs from a panel including less sensitive anticancer drugs [6–7]. Similarly, any anticancer drugs tested must be administered in at least two dosages in drug sensitivity testing. Otherwise, false positive or false negative data may be obtained. In the same way, if we notice, analyze and adhere to all experimental details of drug sensitivity tests, the real drug response to a tumor can easily be obtained and test success can be expected.

In vitro drug sensitivity tests are preferable to *in vivo* drug sensitivity tests, owing to smaller labor requirements and greater technical feasibility, and they are currently more popular than *in vivo* ones. Comparing the two methods, *in vivo* tests often require longer experimental duration, delaying the production of data, and are technically more difficult to handle. Transplantation success rates in both *in vivo* and *in vitro* methods have increased from the initial 25–45% to more than 50%, especially for *in vitro* systems. *In vivo* methods commonly show no obvious advantage over *in vitro* methods in clinical practice. *In vitro* methods can be used to evaluate greater numbers of drugs in a single test, as well as requiring much less labor and taking less time. Since only 2 to 3 drugs are routinely in one *in vivo* test, the number of drug groups compared in such a test is small, markedly diminishing the value of the test for drug selection. From a theoretical standpoint, the quality of treatment is likely to be higher when the range of drugs available for selection is greater. *In vitro* drug sensitivity testing seems advantageous over *in vivo* methods in this respect. Some *in vitro* techniques, such as the ATP-tumor chemosensitivity assay, can evaluate more than 10 anticancer drugs in a single test [11–12]. To address the commonly occurring problems of false-positive or false-negative data, it is advisable to examine more than two concentrations of each drug. It can be even better if dose-response relationships are available and observed [6–7]. More importantly, *in vitro* methods can be used for blood samples from leukemic patients; in contrast, only solid tumor material surgically removed from patients is appropriate for *in vivo* tests. It should also be mentioned that a combination of *in vivo* and *in vitro* methods is presumed to be more useful because the two approaches may provide complementary data.

2.5.2 Induction of multi-drug resistance (MDR) in tumor cells

Induction of MDR in tumor cells often causes conventional chemotherapy to fail. The longer a chemotherapy regime takes, the more likely it is that MDR might be induced in tumor cells. After the induction of MDR in tumor cells, there is no difference between conventional chemotherapy and drug selection by drug sensitivity testing. All that can be done is to add some drug export channel inhibitors to offset the outflow of anticancer drugs in MDR-induced cancer tissues.

2.5.3 No targeting of metastatic cells

90% of cancer patients die of cancer metastasis [21–22]. However, drug sensitivity testing is commonly employed to test drug response to the primary tumor. The failure to specifically target a metastatic tumor makes chemotherapy less beneficial to patients' survival. Individualized cancer chemotherapy specifically targeting neoplasm metastasis is beginning to be in high demand [23–24], especially in late-stage cancer patients with formed metastatic foci (see chapter 5).

These three possible reasons might jointly affect the therapeutic outcomes of chemotherapy regardless of the use of drug sensitivity tests.

2.6 Cytotoxic and cytostatic anti-cancer drugs?

Most anticancer drugs can be divided into two categories: cytotoxic and cytostatic [25]. Cytotoxic anticancer drugs often exhibit strong anticancer effects in drug sensitivity tests or in clinical situations when they are initially used. However, they easily induce multidrug resistance (MDR) and are often useless in terms of a patient's survival benefits. Cytostatic anticancer drugs, which mainly inhibit tumor growth by targeting tumorigenic molecules, show low sensitivity rates in drug sensitivity tests. However, they show better survival benefits than cytotoxic drugs if they are well matched. Therefore, it is optimal to utilize both cytotoxic and cytostatic drugs in a single patient in order to target both tumor growth and metastasis and prolong patients' survival. It is therefore appropriate to predict the response of cytotoxic anticancer drugs to tumors using drug sensitivity tests and to obtain the response information of cytostatic anticancer drugs to tumors from detecting cancer biomarkers or cancer bioinformatics (see chapter 3).

The less than optimal performances of cytotoxic anticancer drugs in patients result mainly from the induction of MDR. Different cytotoxic anticancer drugs often show cross-resistance. For example, it has been reported that a neoplasm tissue that induces resistance to doxorubicin may also induce resistance to other cytotoxic anticancer drugs [26]. This issue should be considered in drug sensitivity tests. When such tests are used, patients benefit by avoiding ineffective anticancer drugs in a trial, reducing hemotoxicity and drug expenditure. The ineffective drugs can also induce cross-resistance, treatment delays and unnecessary treatment-related morbidity and mortality [6–7].

2.7 Conclusion

Drug sensitivity testing is the earliest type of ICC strategy. Most drug sensitivity testing is easy to handle and can be performed in a general hospital. It could be matured by integrating modern ideas and techniques. More advanced drug sensitivity testing methods can be used to select better matched anticancer drugs and to identify correct drug concentrations and less costly performance protocols for cancer patients. Present drug sensitivity testing methods are less effective for choosing the best-matched cytostatic drugs. They should be integrated with other types of ICC strategies.

With the advent of other ICC strategies or the development of more selective anticancer or antimetastatic drugs, the disadvantages of drug sensitivity testing will be reduced or even eliminated. Cancer patients will benefit. We must update and streamline drug sensitivity tests in order eventually to develop effective practical clinical trials.

References

[1] M.M. Black, F.D. Speer, Further observations on the effects of cancer chemotherapeutic agents on the in vitro dehydrogenase activity of cancer tissue, J. Natl. Cancer Inst. 14 (5) (1954) 1147–1158.

[2] J.C. Wright, J.P. Cobb, S.L. Gumport, F.M. Golomb, D. Safadi, Investigation of the relation between clinical and tissue-culture response to chemotherapeutic agents on human cancer, N. Eng. J. Med. 257 (25) (1957) 1207–1211.

[3] A.W. Hamburger, S.E. Salmon, Primary bioassay of human tumor stem cells, Science 197 (4302) (1977) 461–463 (Washington DC).

[4] S.E. Salmon, A.W. Hamburger, B. Soehnlen, B.G.M. Durie, D.S. Alberts, T.E. Moon, Quantitation of differential sensitivity of human-tumor stem cells to anticancer drugs, N. Eng. J. Med. 298 (1978) 1321–1327.

[5] A. Bogden, A rapid screening method for testing chemotherapeutic agents against human tumour xenografts, in: D.O.A. Houchens (Ed.), Proceedings of the Symposium of the use of Athymic (Nude) Mice in Cancer Research, Gustav Fischer Inc, New York, NY, 1978, pp. 231–250.

[6] D.Y. Lu, X.L. Chen, J. Ding, Individualized cancer chemotherapy integrating drug sensitivity tests, pathological profile analysis and computational coordination-an effective strategy to improve clinical treatment, Med. Hypotheses 66 (1) (2006) 45–51.

[7] D.Y. Lu, T.R. Lu, X.L. Chen, J. Ding, Individualized cancer chemotherapy, in: M.M. Shoja, P.S. Agutter, R.S. Tubbs, M. Ghanei, K. Ghabili et al. (Eds.), Hypotheses in Clinical Medicine, Nova Science Publishers, Hauppage, NY, 2012. chapter 13.

[8] H. Morioka, et al., In vitro chemosensitivity of human soft tissue sarcoma, Anticancer Res. 21 (6A) (2001) 4147–4151.

[9] H. Tanino, et al., Acquisition of multidrug resistance in recurrent breast cancer demonstrated by the histoculture drug response assay, Anticancer Res. 21 (6A) (2001) 4083–4086.

[10] R.B. Ness, S.R. Wisniewski, H. Eng, W. Christopherson, Cell viability assay for drug testing in ovarian cancer: in vitro kill versus clinical response, Anticancer Res. 22 (2B) (2002) 1145–1149.

[11] H. Kawamura, K. Ikeda, I. Takiyama, M. Terashima, The usefulness of the ATP assay with serum-free culture for chemosensitivity testing of gastrointestinal cancer, Eur. J. Cancer 33 (6) (1997) 960–966.

[12] C.M. Kurbacher, et al., Use of an ex vivo ATP luminescence assay to direct chemotherapy for recurrent ovarian cancer, Anticancer Drugs 9 (1) (1998) 51–57.

[13] E. Ulukaya, Drug response assay: an increasing trend in designation of tailored-chemotherapy for more rational management of cancer patients, Adv. Mol. Med. 2 (2) (2006) 53–58.

[14] Y. Takamura, et al., Prediction of chemotherapeutic response by collagen gel droplet embedded culture-drug sensitivity test in human breast cancers, Int. J. Cancer 98 (3) (2002) 450–455.

[15] T. Kondo, T. Imamura, H. Ichihashi, In vitro test for sensitivity of tumor to carcinostatic agents, Gann 57 (2) (1966) 113–121.

[16] J.S. Yakisich, Challenges and limitations of targeting cancer stem cells and/or the tumor microenvironment, Drugs Ther. Stud. 2 (2012) e10.
[17] S. Aamdal, O. Fodstad, J.M. Nesland, A. Pihl, Characteristics of human tumour xenografts transplanted under the subrenal capsule of immunocompetent mice, Br. J. Cancer 51 (3) (1985) 347–356.
[18] D. Cunningham, et al., The 6 day subrenal capsule assay is of no value with primary surgical explants from gastric cancer, Br. J. Cancer 54 (3) (1986) 519–523.
[19] F.A. Levi, et al., A four-day subrenal capsule assay for testing the effectiveness of anticancer drugs against human tumors, Cancer Res. 44 (6) (1984) 2660–2667.
[20] D.Y. Lu, et al., Similarity of drug sensitivity test results on human pulmonary adenocarcinoma xenografts transplanted under the subrenal capsules between normal immunocompetent and immunodeficient athymic mice, Int. J. Pharm. Ther. 1 (1) (2010) 106–109.
[21] D.Y. Lu, T.R. Lu, S. Cao, Cancer metastases and clinical therapies, Cell. Dev. Biol. 1 (4) (2012) e110.
[22] S. Valastyan, R.A. Weinberg, Tumor metastasis: molecular insights and evolving paradigms, Cell 147 (2) (2011) 275–292.
[23] D.Y. Lu, T.R. Lu, H.Y. Wu, New insights into individualized antimetastatic therapy, Adv. Tech. Biol. Med. 1 (1) (2013) 106.
[24] D.Y. Lu, T.R. Lu, H.Y. Wu, S. Cao, Cancer metastases treatment, Curr. Drug Ther. 8 (1) (2013) 24–29.
[25] A.W. Millar, K.P. Lynch, Rethinking clinical trials for cytostatic drugs, Nature Rev. Cancer 3 (7) (2003) 540–545.
[26] T. Efferth, V.B. Konkimalla, Y.F. Wang, et al., Prediction of broad spectrum resistance of tumors towards anticancer drugs, Clin. Cancer Res. 14 (2008) 2405–2412.

Individualized cancer chemotherapy via cancer biomarkers or bioinformatics detection

3

3.1 Cancer biomarkers and cancer bioinformatics for ICC [1–3]

3.1.1 Background

Cancer is a disease of genetic alterations or abnormalities. The best therapeutic approaches should target these genetic alterations and abnormalities. However, different cancers are caused by different genetic abnormalities, such as mutation, translocation, deletion, insertion or replication, etc. Thus, before an appropriate therapy can be initiated, it is necessary to know the exact genetic alterations and abnormalities of a specific cancer in clinics [1–7]. Various molecules have been widely reported to have diagnostic and / or prognostic value in cancer patients. Such molecules range from immunoregulatory [8] and inflammatory factors (interleukins and cytokines) and signal transduction regulators (tyrosine kinase, cycloxygenase-2, MAPK, etc.) to factors related to tumor pathology (metastases, angiogenesis and apoptosis), such as vascular epithelial growth factor and its receptor (VEGF and VEGFR), epidermal growth factor receptor (EGFR) and fibrinogen [9]. These biological molecules can be altered or abnormal forms of a genome or molecules such as promote pathogenesis of tumor growth or metastases. These pathogenic biomarkers in tumors are specific targets for drug antagonism or disruption. It has been shown that in patients who have elevated plasma levels of tumorigenic molecules but lack grossly recognizable tumors, the tumorigenic factor levels return to normal following targeted chemotherapy [3]. Small tumor nodules (diameter less than 0.3 mm) are more sensitive to drugs and therefore much better therapeutic outcomes are expected. Last 20 years, this world has witnessed the initiation and rapid progression of bioinformatics study. Cancer bioinformatics study is one of such important omics branches for clinical applications. Same as other biological techniques or systems, bioinformatics are not omni-potent. They have their own limits and shortcomings now. This paragraph will offer a panorama of bioinformatics in cancer researches and clinical applications—a mostly developed area of modern cancer therapy and ICC.

3.1.2 Utilizations in cancer treatment

Before initiating monotherapy (treatment with monoclonal antibodies) or any other type of cytostatic anticancer drug therapies or biotherapies, ideally one should know the levels of their targeted antigens or receptors in tumors in order to provide a rational basis for treatments. Tumor biomarker detection methods normally require surgical samples and can also be conducted without fresh tumor samples as a prerequisite. Routine blood and tumor sample tests can be useful in leukemia patients. With the increasing development of highly selective drugs (cytostatic anticancer drugs or biotherapies), cancer patients can be treated with more targeted cytostatic anticancer agents or biotherapies chosen by reference only to pathophysiological data (cancer biomarkers) without using drug sensitivity tests. Examples of successes include fluoropyrimidine-based chemotherapy for metastatic colon cancers over-expressing dihydropyrimidine dehydrogenase and thymidylate synthase, and treatment of the deadliest lung cancers resulting from EGFR mutation with a specific kinase inhibitor, Iressa [3].

3.2 Seeing is predicting

In early stages, cancer biomarker detection is focused on one or several pathogenic molecules (commonly protein or glycol-protein). Targeted monoclonal antibodies or other cytostatic anticancer drugs are prescribed for patients with high levels of cancer biomarkers. From recently, high-throughput cancer bioinformatics methods are used to identify a spectrum of cancer biomarkers, including tumorigenic initiators and promoters, and further deciding which cytostatic anticancer drugs are most likely to target these neoplasm tissues [2–7]. Since tumors are progressive pathogenesis processes with more than a hundred genetic changes accumulating in a single cell [10–11], high-throughput methods are needed to identify or pinpoint these underlying multigenic abnormalities. The multidisciplinary nature of bioinformatics makes it more costly and the assistant tools for deciphering cancer bioinformatics data are harder to handle. Individualized treatment based on the use of cancer bioinformatics for detecting and understanding molecular and genetic variation is a modern strategy. Individualized cancer chemotherapy might range from the detection of just one or two protein or glycoprotein biomarkers to high-throughput genetic and molecular bioinformatics. It relies on real clinical situations and cost-effectiveness considerations.

Cancers have different etiological bases but share the same pathological characteristic of unlimited growth. They result from genetic malfunction and molecular disturbances. Using the cancer genome to help understand the cause of cancer and variable response to drugs will be its most important application in medicine [12]. More than a thousand types of genetic abnormality can result in more than one hundred different tumor types. More than one hundred different anticancer drugs are available for treatment of different cancer categories and types. Even with a certain tumor type, such as lung cancer or mammary cancer, the responses to the same anticancer drugs may vary from patient to patient. Bioinformatics is a genomics-based approach and provides a variety of techniques for analyzing abnormalities of DNA, RNA, proteins and glycoligands as a whole in tumors. In the earliest era of the use of biomarkers in bioinformatics evaluations, clinical cancer practice was to provide patients' prognoses [13] or classify tumor origins [14]. Presently and in future, the best use of biomarkers or bioinformatics for predicting anticancer drug responses is to decide on monotherapy (treatment of cancer patients with monoclonal antibodies) or other biotherapeutic means, such as therapeutic vaccines. In early-stage cancer patients, if a tumorigenic biomarker in a tumor tissue has been detected at an abnormally high level, it is reasonable to assume that the monoclonal antibodies specifically targeting this biomarker will be ideally effective against this tumor. Numerous reports have addressed this issue and some successful results have been obtained [15–18]. On the other hand, the monoclonal antibodies are very expensive and thousands of US dollars can be spent on drugs in a single therapeutic cycle. Usually, only a few months of survival is all the benefit that can be expected in late-stage cancer patients. The short-term survival benefits of therapeutic antibodies might be caused by the production of human immune responses to these antibodies [19]. In some early-stage cancer patients, marked therapeutic outcomes have frequently been seen. Some authors have reported no survival benefit after monotherapy. This is only a hypothesis, as we do not clearly detect abnormal cancer biomarkers [20–21].

3.3 New challenges

Extrapolating exact alleles of genetic alteration or abnormalities in cancer cells is no easy task. It involves the detection of DNA, RNA, protein and glycoprotein. In the detection of proteins or glycoproteins, the results are straightforward. In the detection of oncogenomic information, however, the extrapolation is relatively complicated. A genome is more than a bundle of genes. Apart from protein-encoding regions, non-protein-encoding regions and repetitive DNA are also present in the human genome [22]. It and the oncogenome contain non-coding RNA genes, regulatory sequences, structural motifs; they maintain short-range and long-range spatial organization of sequences; and also contain evolutionary information [23]. Thus the extrapolation of genetic abnormalities from a tumor tissue calls for high technology and revolutionary knowledge and calculating systems. The more we understand the human genome, the more correct genetic information and accurate therapeutic targets we can choose from, and optimal clinical outcomes can be achieved in future by using targeted anticancer or antimetastatic drugs.

3.4 Discussion

Bioinformatics methods, with state-of-the-art technology and equipment, are important for identifying the original and causative biomarkers in any individualized chemotherapy [3–7]. To attain this goal, many more basic and clinical investigations are needed to establish good routines and paradigms for clinical practitioners to follow. These routines and paradigms need to be easy to handle, less costly, high-throughput, and as effective as possible. Currently, there are many different bioinformatics techniques to select overall biomarker changes amongst tumor cells and no single technique seems advantageous over the rest. It is recommended that an international committee should be encouraged to work on this issue, and standard chips or techniques be designed and made uniform by manufacturers in order to safeguard the quality and cost of investigations in future [3].

3.5 Other considerations

Apart from monotherapy, some small-molecular cytostatic anticancer drugs can also be chosen by consulting biomarker information. Selecting this type of anticancer or antimetastatic drug chemotherapy depends on implementing a sophisticated calculating system to analyze high-throughput data. The exact tumorigenic pathways that a drug inhibits or blocks and the cost of therapies need to be understood [24]. It must also be known how far a drug acts and what possible toxicities it has, so the balance between efficacy and risk can be evaluated [25], and whether it is cost-effective in the therapeutic application of detecting cancer biomarkers [6,26]. This requires the retrieval, interpretation and meta-analysis of clinical or pharmacogenetics data.

A good therapeutic schedule can be achieved by detecting human cancer bio-markers. Forexample, treatment of metastatic breast cancer with trastuzumab should be based on observing that the metastatic breast cancer is positive in HER2. Though the trastuzumab (an antibody to HER2) is very expensive, the survival benefit is considerably improved compared with that ensuing from other types of antibodies in HER2-positive metastatic breast cancers. However, if the metastatic breast cancer is negative in HER2, the therapeutic benefits of trastuzumab will be low [27].

3.6 Mathematical modeling and computational networks as assistant systems

Mathematics is becoming increasingly pervasive in various fields of biology and medicine [28–31]. Mathematical modeling and computational networks are powerful tools for helping decision-making and for defining and meeting the ultimate goals of ICC. These tools will help to select crucial targets from the wealth of tumorigenic factors and bioinformatics data, weigh the importance of each variable and finally coordinate and decide matched drugs to rectify the escalated biomarkers in tumors. Generally, mathematical techniques can be used to coordinate treatment schedules and integrate multi-variant pathological data. A mathematical approach that helps us to optimize therapeutic efficiency will become an indispensable part of ICC in future. Currently, mathematical studies for cancer chemotherapy focus largely on the requisite plasma drug concentration and cost-effectiveness in terms of the controlling budget, but mathematical approaches can potentially do far more than that. As quantitative data are always superior to qualitative descriptions for decision-making, mathematical methods will be used in the future to perform more quantitative calculations than ever before and handle and treat sophisticated bioinformatics data. The current and future systems of mathematics in ICC must be built around processing and extracting drug-sensitivity-testing data and / or establishing biomarker-orientated therapy with long-term follow-up of the patient's survival and quality of life by using ICC strategies for predicting anticancer drug responses.

3.7 Finding tumorigenic markers from the genome to predict anticancer drug responses

Finding tumorigenic markers from tumor tissue genomes is an important statistical and mathematical challenge in ICC. It is known that there are about 35,000 genes in a normal human cell. Each individual has a distinctive genetic makeup, and the expression of some of the 35,000 genes will be higher or lower in a tumor cell than in normal cells. Only one or two of them are likely to be the original genetic abnormalities that caused tumorigenesis and led to further and more widespread abnormalities of gene expression [3,9,32]. When the genetic status of a tumor is assessed, only an average or overall picture of gene expression is obtained. In most cancer cells, there are many alterative genetic alleles. After detection of all alterative cancer biomarkers, we can use different cytostatic anticancer drug combinations directly targeting all the altered cancer biomarkers. And the original genetic abnormalities have to be extracted from this wealth of data using mathematical procedures. Currently, usually only a few cancer biomarkers are detected in routine hospital procedures. Hence, the origin of a tumor is unlikely to be identified by this hospital routine. More comprehensive approaches to mapping the genetic polymorphisms and cytological levels of biomarkers, as well as the application of increasingly sophisticated mathematical means, will be required to pinpoint the real culprit from the wealth of bioinformatics data in order to optimize the efficacy of anticancer drugs. The mathematical treatment for deriving genetic, RNA and protein information and relationships between cancer bioinformatics and the prediction of drug responses will be desired or indispensable parts of future ICC strategies. Very useful computer software that supports automatic prediction of drug responses may be developed and formally used in hospitals in the future.

3.8 Future directions

Four types of clinical investigations will help to perfect the cancer biomarker-based ICC strategy:

1. validating and pinpointing the cancer biomarkers or bioinformatics from tumor samples, deducing which targeted cytostatic anticancer drugs or biotherapies might be most effective, and establishing the relationship between individual biomarker changes and the effectiveness of relevant anticancer drugs;
2. technical improvements in the analytical capacity for biomarker detection, decreasing the cost of such detection per unit, and finally validation and identification of key cancer biomarkers from the whole genome by mathematical means;
3. evaluation and prediction of tumor responses to each anticancer drug in different pathological conditions with varying genetic abnormalities; and finally
4. design of a genetic rectification system targeted at the real-time situations of patients [1,3].

Individualized cancer chemotherapy, developed by detecting cancer biomarkers or bioinformatics is a new and modern method compared with drug sensitivity tests and has great potential. It is currently underestimated. Compared to the use of therapeutic anticancer drugs and taking into account the cost of residence in hospital (more than $10,000), the cost of cancer biomarker detection is relatively low ($100-5000). It is cost-effective for most early-stage cancer patients [6,26–27]. With the development of biological detecting techniques, individualized cancer chemotherapy by means of the detection of cancer biomarkers or bioinformatics is a way complementary to drug sensitivity testing and anticancer drug pharmacogenetics. The benefits to chemotherapy are obvious and straightforward. This will be the fastest-growing area of ICC in future. However, individualized cancer chemotherapy developed by detecting cancer biomarkers or bioinformatics is also designed for primary tumors. Biomarkers relating to tumor metastases must be analyzed [2] and antimetastatic drugs also administered if there is a strong likelihood of tumor metastasis.

References

[1] D.Y. Lu, X.L. Chen, J. Ding, Individualized cancer chemotherapy integrating drug sensitivity tests, pathological profile analysis and computational coordination-an effective strategy to improve clinical treatment, Med. Hypotheses 66 (1) (2006) 45–51.

[2] D.Y. Lu, T.R. Lu, S. Cao, Individualized cancer chemotherapy by detecting cancer biomarkers, Metabolomics 2 (5) (2012) e121.

[3] D.Y. Lu, T.R. Lu, X.L. Chen, J. Ding, Individualized cancer chemotherapy, in: M.M. Shoja, P.S. Agutter, R.S. Tubbs, M. Ghanei, K. Ghabili et al. (Eds.), Hypotheses in Clinical Medicine, Nova Science Publishers, Hauppage, NY, 2012. chapter 13.

[4] W.S. Dalton, S.H. Friend, Cancer biomarkers--an invitation to the table, Science 312 (5777) (2006) 1165–1168.

[5] A. Ocana, A. Pandiella, Personalized therapies in the cancer “omics” era, Mol. Cancer 9 (2010) 202.

[6] V.P. Retèl, M.A. Joore, M. Knauer, S.C. Linn, M. Hauptmann, et al., Cost-effectiveness of the 70-gene signature versus st. gallen guidelines and adjuvant online for early breast cancer, Eur. J. Cancer 46 (8) (2010) 1382–1391.

[7] B. Stransky, P. Galante, Application of bioinformatics in cancer research, in: W.C.S. Cho (Ed.), An OMICS Perspective on Cancer Research, 12, Springer, Dordrecht, NL, 2010, pp. 211–233.

[8] B.M. Olson, D.G. McNeel, Monitoring regulatory immune responses tumor immunotherapy clinical trials, Frontiers Oncol. 3 (2013) 109.

[9] D. Hanahan, R.A. Weinberg, The hallmarks of cancer, Cell 100 (1) (2000) 57–70.

[10] D.L. Stoler, N. Chen, M. Basik, M.S. Kahlenberg, M.A. Rodriguez-Bigas, et al., The onset and extent of genomic instability in sporadic colorectal tumor progression, Proc. Natl. Acad. Sci. 96 (26) (1999) 15121–15126.

[11] C.V. Jongeneel, C. Isseli, B. Stevenson, G. J. Riggins, A. Lal, et al., Comprehensive sampling of gene expression in human cell lines with massively parallel signature sequencing, Proc. Natl. Acad. Sci. 100 (8) (2003) 4702–4705.

[12] R.L. Strausberg, A.J.G. Simpson, L.J. Old, G.J. Riggins, Oncogenomics and the development of new cancer therapies, Nature 429 (2004) 469–474.

[13] M.J. Van de Vijer, Y.D. He, L. Van't Veer, et al., A gene-expression signature as a predictor of survival in breast cancer, N. Engl. J. Med. 347 (2002) 1999–2009.

[14] G.J. Gordon, R.V. Jensen, L.L. Hsaio, S.R. Gullans, J.E. Blumenstock, et al., Translation of microarray data into clinically relevant cancer diagnostic tests using gene expression ratios in lung cancer and mesothelioma, Cancer Res. 62 (17) (2002) 4963–4967.
[15] V. Diehl, Hodgkin's disease from pathology specimen to cure, N. Engl. J. Med. 357 (2007) 1968–1971.
[16] C.E. Geyer, J. Forster, D. Lindquist, S. Chan, G. Romieu, et al., Lapatinib plus capecitabine for her2-positive advanced breast cancer, N. Engl. J. Med. 355 (2006) 2733–2743.
[17] J.B. Vermorken, R. Mesia, F. Rivera, E. Remenar, A. Kawecki, S. Rottey, et al., Platinum-based chemotherapy plus cetuximab in head and neck cancer, N. Engl. J. Med. 359 (2008) 1116–1127.
[18] A. Younes, N.L. Bartlett, J.P. Leonard, D.A. Kennedy, C.M. Lynch, et al., Brentuximab vedotin (SGN-35) for relapsed CD30-positive lymphomas, N. Engl. J. Med. 363 (2010) 1812–1821.
[19] C. Warnke, C. Hermanrud, M. Lundkvist, A. Fogdell-Hahn, Anti-drug antibodies, Drugs Ther. Stud. 2 (1) (2012) e11.
[20] J. Tol, M. Koopman, A. Cats, C.J. Rodenburg, G.J.M. Creemers, et al., Chemotherapy, bevacizumab, and cetuximab in metastatic colorectal cancer, N. Engl. J. Med. 360 (2009) 563–572.
[21] K. Miller, M. Wang, J. Gralow, M. Dickler, M. Cobleigh, et al., Paclitaxel plus bevacizumab versus paclitaxel alone for metastatic breast cancer, N. Engl. J. Med. 357 (2007) 2666–2676.
[22] D.R. Bentley, Genomes for medicine, Nature 429 (2004) 440–445.
[23] T.S. Foster, et al., The economic burden of metastatic breast cancer: a systematic review of literature from developed countries, Cancer Treatment Rev. 37 (6) (2011) 405–415.
[24] Z.A. Knight, K.M. Shokat, Chemical genetics: where genetics and pharmacology meet, Cell 128 (3) (2007) 425–430.
[25] D.Y. Lu, T.R. Lu, J. Ding, Employing new mathematical models and equations to evaluate risk-benefit criteria of clinical therapeutics, Online J. Biol. Sci. 7 (1) (2007) 1–2.
[26] V.P. Retèl, M.A. Joore, M. Knauer, S.C. Linn, M. Hauptmann, et al., Cost-effectiveness of the 70-gene signature versus St. Gallen guidelines and adjuvant online for early breast cancer, Eur. J. Cancer 46 (8) (2010) 1382–1391.
[27] J.L. Lesnock, C. Farris, T.C. Krivak, K.J. Smith, M. Markman, Consolidation paclitaxel is more cost-effective than bevacizumab following upfront treatment of advanced epithelial ovarian cancer, Gynecol. Oncol. 122 (3) (2011) 473–478.
[28] E. Pennisi, Tracing life's circuitry, Science 302 (5651) (2003) 1646–1649.
[29] N. Friedman, Inferring cellular networks using probabilistic graphical models, Science 303 (5659) (2004) 799–805.
[30] J. Hoh, J. Ott, Mathematical multi-locus approaches to localizing complex human trait genes, Nature Rev. Genet. 4 (9) (2003) 701–709.
[31] P.Z. Hu, G. Bader, D.A. Wigle, A. Emili, Computational prediction of cancer-gene function, Nature Rev. Cancer 7 (2007) 23–34.
[32] P.C. Nowell, The clonal evolution of tumor cell populations, Science 194 (4260) (1976) 23–28 (Washington DC).

Pharmacogenetics

4

4.1 Background

In the opening years of this millennium, the systematic study of pharmacogenetics has been intensified. People began to understand that most drugs undergo structural modification under the action of hepatic or other organ metabolism enzymes in human bodies, with activation or inactivation of drugs [1–3]. Some drug modifications can produce anticancer metabolites or inactivate active drugs or metabolites into non-active metabolites. The percentage proportion of these active to inactive drug metabolites is decided or determined by inherent genetic conditions in patients. It is known that plasma concentrations, drug responses and toxicities of anticancer drugs can vary more than tenfold among different tumor tissues or patients who are given the same dosages of anticancer drugs in clinics because of genetic variations or genetic polymorphisms in drug metabolism enzymes or cancer biomarkers. The purpose of pharmacogenetics is to predict the fraction of active or inactive metabolites, the required dosage of a drug, and the possible sensitivity of tumors to anticancer or antimetastatic drugs by analyzing the genetic status of the drug metabolism enzymes or targeted cancer molecules in cancer patients, or targeting the biomarker status of the cancer tissues [4–7]. Overall, pharmacogenetics or pharmacogenomics is an effort to maximize efficacy and minimize toxicities of drugs in patients. "Pharmacogenetics or Pharmacogenomics" (PG) represents the study of human genetic factors affecting drug toxicities or responses in treated patients. Despite of human genetic or genomic information for forecasting disease risk, optimizing treatment agents or dosing regimens, predictions of drug toxicities and responses to cancer growth or dissemination to remote sites, something uniqueness relating to anticancer therapy PG needs to be specially noticed. Similarities and differences between cancer therapy PG and other disease therapy PG are reiterated herein and many cancer therapy PG protocols or applications need to be improved in future.

4.2 Introduction

The term "pharmacogenetics," denoting the study of genetic factors that influence response to drugs and chemicals, was first coined in 1959 [8]. Since the beginning of this millennium, large-scale human genetic studies have been transforming pharmacogenetics or pharmacogenomics into potential clinical disciplines. Many effective drugs, including anticancer drugs, have been systematically studied in different patients and different tumor categories. Patients' genetic information has been used in forecasting disease risk, choosing treatment agents and drug dosage.

Pharmacogenetics or pharmacogenomics detects genetic information such as single nucleotide polymorphisms (SNP) of human metabolism enzymes, haplotypes, microsatellites or simple sequence repeats, insertion and / or deletion, copy number variations and aneupoidy of human metabolism enzymes and tumor tissues.

There are two basic models of anticancer drug pharmacogenomics:

(i) control and optimization of the concentrations of active anticancer drugs or metabolites;
(ii) pharmacogenetic study of anticancer or antimetastatic drugs targeting genes (tumor tissues or metastatic foci).

4.2.1 *Control the concentrations of active anticancer drugs*

There are a number of different metabolites of anticancer drugs in human blood or plasma. They are determined by human metabolizing enzymes. Many different human metabolizing enzymes determine the metabolisms of different anticancer drugs (Figure 4.1). If one human metabolizing enzyme is affected by genetic polymorphism, some anticancer prodrugs cannot produce enough active anticancer drug metabolites. Then the tumor inhibition of anticancer drugs will be reduced. On the other hand, active anticancer drugs may be more quickly detoxicated or excreted by human metabolizing enzymes. If these human metabolizing enzymes are inactivated by the genetic polymorphism of enzyme genes, the active anticancer drugs will be more intensively accumulated in blood and plasma in human bodies. These patients will show the strong toxicity of anticancer drugs, some of them even life-threatening. (See Figure 4.2.) This is the major thrust of anticancer drug pharmacogenetics [4–7].

4.2.2 Pharmacogenetic study of anticancer or antimetastatic drugs targeting genes

Pharmacogenetic study of drugs targeting genes is another aspect of anticancer drug individualized therapy (Figure 4.3). Anticancer drugs exhibit anticancer activity by inhibiting targeted cancer genes or molecules. If these targeted genes or molecules are influenced by human genetic polymorphism, such as SNP, a drug's response to the genes will change greatly. These targeted cancer molecules or genes can be all oncogenic or metastatic related genes or molecules.

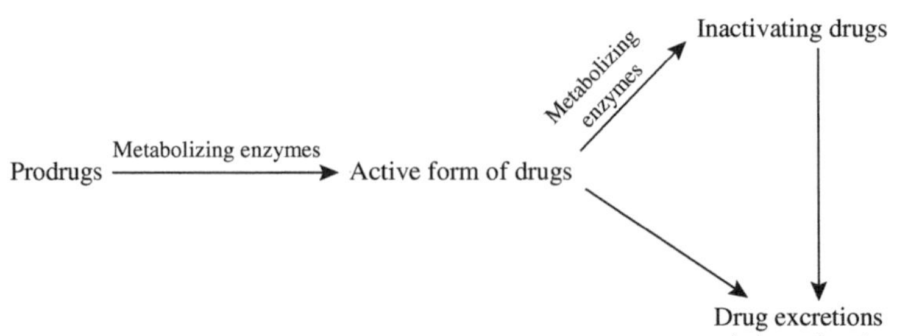

Figure 4.1 The relationship between drug concentration and polymorphism of metabolizing enzymes.

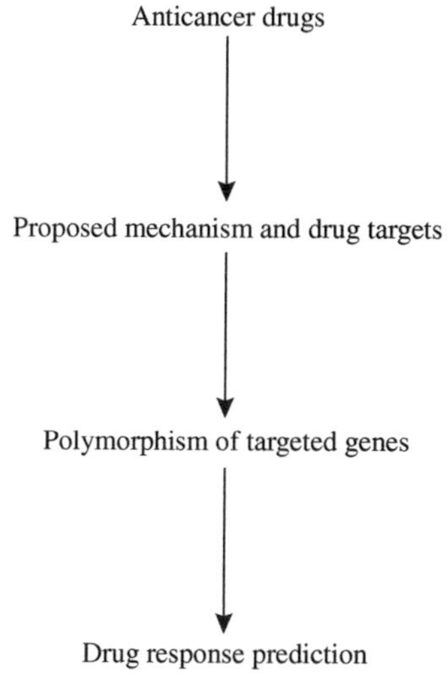

Figure 4.2 General scheme of drug response prediction in pharmacogenetics study.

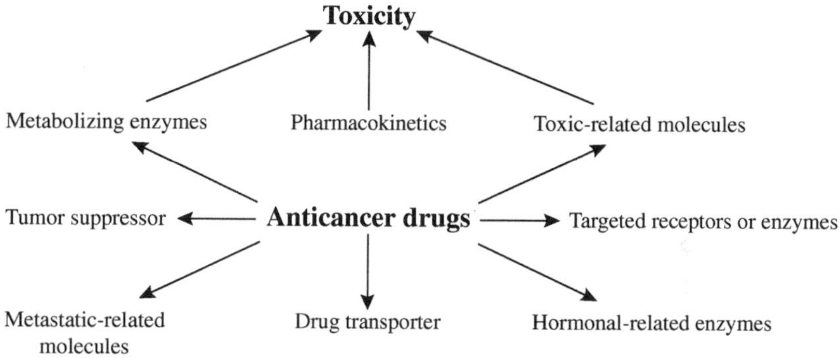

Figure 4.3 The field of pharmacogenetics in individualized cancer chemotherapy.

Since the number of genes or molecules with oncogenic or metastatic associations is extremely large, it is very hard to decide which genes or molecules to detect first. Other ICC strategies might be better suited for drug choice and then genes or molecules targeted by the drugs can be detected.

4.3 Architectural framework of an anticancer drug pharmacogenetics or pharmacogenomics study

4.3.1 Problems of cancer therapy

The major obstacles arising in cancer chemotherapy are the development of drug resistance and the severe side effects and tumor metastasis. Due to the modest tumor specificity of many anticancer drugs, normal tissues are also damaged. This prevents the application of doses sufficiently high to eradicate less sensitive tumor cell populations.

Thereby, tumors develop drug resistance, leading to treatment failure and fatal consequences for patients. Apart from this, cancer metastasis is responsible for 90% of cancer deaths. Pharmacogenetics applications in cancers require analysis of the genetic status of individual patients for each drug to predict if this drug is highly active or highly toxic in a given individual. Large inter-individual variation is observed in both the response and the toxicity associated with anticancer therapy (Figure 4.3).

Pharmacogenetics or pharmacogenomics first determines the role of genetics in drug toxicity or responses. It often comes from clinical evidence or experience or hypothesis-driven systematic studies. Then comes screening and identification of genetic markers. After enough clinical data is accumulated, the computation, validation and definition of these clinical data of genetic markers, new knowledge and clinical pharmacogenetics practice can be initiated; next, clinical utility, assessment and transforming new knowledge into application [7].

The overall theme of pharmacogenetics is 'the right drug for the right patient'. It includes detection of polymorphism in the following genes [5]:

1. Upstream mechanisms
   Drug transporters (drug resistance);
   Drug-metabolizing phase I enzymes (CYP subfamily enzymes) (prodrug to active metabolites or inactivation of drugs);
   Drug-metabolizing phase II enzymes (other than CYP enzymes) (inactivation of anticancer drugs).
2. Drug target interactions
   DNA biosynthesis and metabolism (alkalating agents and platinum drugs);
   DNA repair mechanisms (toxicity or resistance of drugs);
   Cell signal receptors;
   Mitotic spindles (possibly provoking drug resistance);
   Hormone-regulated enzyme;
   HIF-related pathways;
   Nuclear-factor-related pathways, etc.
3. Downstream mechanisms; apoptosis genes and chemokines
   Tumor suppressor p53 (drug response or resistance);
   Bcl;
   Fas/CD95/Apo-1;
   PTEN;
   Tumor necrosis factors (TNF) and interleukin 10;
   Interleukin 6, etc.
4. Tumor metastasis-related pathways (drugs targeting neoplasm metastasis)
   MMPs;
   CAM (cell adhesion molecules); integrins, cadherins, selectins, etc.;
   Angiogenesis genes, etc.

4.3.2 General methods and areas of pharmacogenetics

Explanations of polymorphism of key enzymes or molecules for understanding responses or resistance to or toxicity of drugs, or finally understanding drug responses to tumor metastasis.

1. From inactive prodrug to active metabolites
   There is now a steady increase in the numbers of prodrugs marketed, for example, Irinotecan, Topotecan. For these prodrugs, the polymorphisms of drug-metabolizing enzymes can be used to predict the level of active metabolites. Drug-metabolizing enzymes, mainly consisting of different isoforms of cytochrome P450 monoxygenases (CYP) are major constituents of human metabolizing enzymes; if too few active metabolites of drugs are produced, the treatment will probably be less effective. If too many active metabolites of drugs are produced, high toxicity or secondary tumors are possible.
2. Prediction of drug resistance
   One of the thorny problems in cancer chemotherapy is the occurrence of multi-drug resistance (MDR). Now more experiments and increasing clinical evidence suggest that a series of drug transporter molecules, such as ATP-binding cassette transporters (ABC transporters), P-glycoprotein (ABCB1, MDR1), multidrug-resistance-related proteins (MRPs) et al., decide the nature of drug resistance. Thus, detection of genetic polymorphisms of these molecules can enable us to predict whether or not there will be drug resistance. Also, if DNA repair mechanisms are mutated, this will raise or reduce the possibility of drug resistance.
3. Prediction of drug response
   Prediction of drug response is the most important topic in cancer chemotherapy. Several factors can vary drug responses to tumors, including the polymorphism of targeted molecules, of drug-metabolizing enzymes, and of tumor-suppressive molecules. Anticancer drug selection will be based on the detection of polymorphism in drug response genes.
4. Prediction of drug toxicity
   Prediction of drug toxicity relies on both drug-metabolizing enzymes and the organs with potential drug toxicity. For example, if the metabolizing enzyme for a drug is mutated or nullified, the plasma level of the drug will increase and the toxicity of this drug or even the possibility of creating secondary tumors will also increase. Again, when one type of human DNA-repair mechanisms is impaired, the possibility of drug resistance and drug-induced cancer will increase.
5. Prediction of drug response to neoplasm metastases
   Cancer treatment targeting neoplasm metastases is different from treatment targeting a primary tumor (chapter 5). But cancer patients with metastasizing foci often have a small chance of survival. Genetic polymorphism of cancer metastasis-related pathways might be helpful for drug selection and responses in cancer patients with or without metastasis.

4.4 Examples

4.4.1 Toxicity

Platinum agent-induced gastrointestinal toxicity is associated with polymorphism of ERCC1 gene and irinotecan-induced hematologic toxicity is associated with the polymorphism of metabolizing enzyme UGT1A1*28 [9]. A drug can be toxic for different reasons and to multiple organs. This increases the difficulty of pharmacogenomic studies of drug toxicities. So many side effects, if not very severe or not easily defined, are commonly neglected in the study of pharmacogenetics or pharmacogenomics. There is no clear-cut definition of the degrees of toxicity. Whether or not a pharmacogenetic study is used depends on the experience of the doctor and facilities of the hospital.

Thiopurine S-methyltransferase (TPMT) is a metabolizing enzyme that inactivates some active metabolites of anticancer drugs, such as 6-mercaptopurine, azathioprine and 6-thioguanine. Normally, 90% of individuals have high TPMT enzymatic activity. 10% individuals have intermediate TPMT activity. 0.3% of individuals have low or even no detectable TPMT activity. Among TPMT-deficient persons, variations TPMT*2, TPMT*3A and TPMT*3C show 95% TPMT enzyme-activity deficiency. Inability to inactivate active drug metabolites will cause severe, even life-threatening toxicity in patients, [10].

Among these metabolizing enzymes, there are several SNPs in most enzyme genes. These enzyme SNPs vary with ethnic differences. *See Tables 4.1 and 4.2. So in some ethnic groups, there is no need to look for certain SNPs.

Table 4.1 Ethnic frequencies (%) of allelic variants in CYP2B6

Allelic variants	SNP	Caucasian	African American	Asian	Hispanic
CYP2B6*2	C64T	5.3–9.0	0	4.7	
CYP2B6*3	C777A	0.5		0	
CYP2B6*4	A785G	4.0–32.6	16.7	9.3	14.3
CYP2B6*5	C1459T	9.5–13	9.0	1.1	0
CYP2B6*6	G516T A785G	25.6		16.4	
CYP2B6*7	G516T A785G C1459T	0–0.3		0	
CYP2B6*8	A415G	1.0	0	0	0

SNY, single nucleotide polymorphism Ref 6.

Table 4.2 Ethnic frequencies (%) of allelic variants in CYP2C9

Allelic variant	SNP	Caucasians	Africa-American	Asians	Hispanics	Africans
CYP2C9*2	C430T	6.8–13.2	1.0–2.5	0	8.0	
CYP2C9*3	A1075C	4.3–15.9	0.5–1.25	0–2.2	6.0	
CYP2C9*5	C1080G	0	1.7			
CYP2C9*7	C55A					7.1
CYP2C9*8	G449A		6.7			7.1
CYP2C9*9	A752G	0.5	13.3			14.3
CYP2C9*11	C1003T	1				
CYP2C9*12	C1465T	0.5				

SNY, single nucleotide polymorphism Ref 6.

4.5 Discussion

Choice of anticancer drugs is an important aspect of pharmacogenetics studies and applications. Pharmacogenetics can guide us to precisely administer and monitor concentration of specific anticancer drugs in humans. There are many genetic factors that can affect drug toxicities and responses. Pharmacogenetics is the way to effective choice and proper utilization of anticancer drugs.

Pharmacogenetics and pharmacogenomics studies have successfully identified genetic variants that contribute to these variations in susceptibility and toxic response to chemotherapeutics. Though numerous pharmacogenetics or pharmacogenomics studies have been reported, successful clinical applications are very limited. Among these studies, detected genetic variations affecting drug plasma concentration are commonly less dramatic than we have expected, and sometimes contradictory. So a large part of current pharmacogenetics or pharmacogenomics studies is the buildup of a foundation for further effective work and potential clinical applications. This discipline must be taken from the bench to the bedside.

Pharmacogenetics or pharmacogenomics help clinical personnel to know how to use a specific anticancer drug, but pharmacogenetics and pharmacogenomics cannot show why this anticancer drug must be used to target a specific tumor origin. It is drug sensitivity testing, or cancer biomarker detection, that can show which drugs must be used for any specific tumor origin.

There is an imbalance between the rapid development of genotyping technology, the marketing of genetic tests, and the high levels of uncertainty in interpreting clinical significance. More success stories from pharmacogenetics or pharmacogenomics applications are needed. For pharmacogenetics and pharmacogenomics to succeed, greater accumulation of experimental or clinical data is required. Present knowledge of genetic influences on drug response and toxicity does not even amount to a fifth of what we should know. Without enough experimental or clinical data, we cannot build a solid foundation to support real clinical use of anticancer drug pharmacogenetics. We may in time obtain enough genotype-phenotype association or gene-drug relationship information to serve the goal of increasing cancer patients' survival.

But drug responses in humans are often multigenetic, and effectiveness with respect to one gene may imply resistance to other genes, or even trigger multi-drug resistance. So this type of research is still at a preliminary stage and its generally relatively high cost of detection (100-5000 USD) renders it impractical in most clinical circumstances.

Since cancer metastasis is responsible for 90% of cancer patient deaths, more rigorous assessment is urgently needed to determine the clinical significance of genetic polymorphisms of metastatis-related genes or molecules and streamline treatment protocols and optimum patient survival benefits with anticancer or antimetastatic drugs [11–15]. (Chapter 5.)

There is no central dogma of pharmacogenetics or pharmacogenomics studies to follow. All that is needed is intuition, hypothesis-driven data collection and computations. The more we hypothesize and testify that a specific gene works with a specific drug, the more clinical drug sensitivity evidence we may obtain, and the better and more sophisticated the pharmacogenetics and pharmacogenomics information and clinical utilization we can achieve.

References

[1] W.E. Evans, J.A. Johnson, Pharmacogenomics; the inherited basis for interindividual differences in drug response, Annu. Rev. Genomics. Hum. Genet. 2 (2001) 9–39.
[2] W.E. Evans, M.V. Relling, Moving towards individualized medicine with pharmacogenomics, Nature 429 (2004) 464–468.
[3] D.B. Goldstein, S.K. Tate, S.M. Sisodiya, Pharmacogenetics goes genomic, Nat. Rev. Genet. 4 (12) (2003) 937–947.
[4] J.W. Watters, H.L. McLeod, Cancer pharmacogenomics: current and future applications, Biochim. Biophys. Acta 1603 (2) (2003) 99–111.
[5] T. Efferth, M. Volm, Pharmacogenetics for individualized cancer chemotherapy, Pharmacol. Ther. 107 (2) (2005) 155–176.
[6] J.F. Deeken, W.D. Figg, S.E. Bates, A. Sparreboom, Toward individualized treatment: prediction of anticancer drug disposition and toxicity with pharmacogenetics, Anticancer Drugs 18 (2) (2007) 111–126.
[7] R.S. Huang, M.J. Ratain, Pharmacogenetics and pharmacogenomics of anticancer agents, CA. Cancer J. Clin. 59 (1) (2009) 42–55.
[8] U.A. Meyer, Pharmacogenetics – five decades of therapeutic lessons from genetic diversity, Nat. Rev. Genet. 5 (2004) 669–676.
[9] J. Hoskins, et al., UGT1A1*28 genotype and irinotecan-induced neutropenia: dose matters, J. Natl. Cancer Inst. 99 (17) (2007) 1290–1295.
[10] H.L. McLeod, C. Siva, The thiopurine S-methyltransferase gene locus – implications for clinical pharmacogenomics, Pharmacogenomics 3 (1) (2002) 89–98.
[11] L. Liu, M. Sun, D. Song, Z. Wang, The genetic polymorphisms of intercellular cell adhesion molecules and breast cancer susceptibility; a meta-analysis, Mol. Biol. Rep. 40 (2) (2013) 1855–1860.
[12] D.Y. Lu, T.R. Lu, S. Cao, Cancer metastases and clinical Therapies, Cell Dev Biol 1 (4) (2012) e110.
[13] S. Valastyan, R.A. Weinberg, Tumor metastasis: molecular insights and evolving paradigms, Cell 147 (2) (2011) 275–292.
[14] D.Y. Lu, T.R. Lu, H.Y. Wu, New insights into individualized antimetastatic therapy, Adv. Tech. Biol. Med. 1 (1) (2013) 106.
[15] D.Y. Lu, T.R. Lu, H.Y. Wu, S. Cao, Cancer metastases treatment, Curr. Drug Ther. 8 (1) (2013) 24–29.

Individualized antimetastatic therapy [1–2]

5

5.1 Background

Cancer metastasis, as the main cause of death in cancer patients, is the key to averting these deaths. More than 90% of cancer deaths are caused by metastasis. Up to now, treatment of cancer patients is focused mainly on primary tumors and antimetastatic drugs are seen as assistant therapy; as a result, only a few antimetastatic drug types have been licensed. Many individualized cancer chemotherapy methods, such as drug sensitivity tests or pharmacogenomics, are designed to target primary tumors. So far there has been a small improvement in clinical survival rates. Now there seems basically no better option than drugs for antimetastatic treatment, yet cancer metastasis treatment in clinics commonly does not work. Any small breakthrough for antimetastatic therapy will mean substantial clinical achievements in cancer therapy [3]. So, to reiterate, more attention needs to be paid to developing more effective antimetastatic drugs and treating neoplasm metastases according to patients' clinical circumstances, as well as finding effective therapies to combat formed metastatic foci. Since cancer metastasis is the main cause of cancer patients' deaths, antimetastatic treatment studies should play decisive roles for elongation of cancer patients' survival. Past three decades, despite cancer metastatic biological or pathological theories have been proved again and again by new biological techniques, translational or clinical studies against neoplasm metastasis are less fruitful. Facing these challenges, promoting the studies of all these new attempts might change the landscape of metastasis treatments.

5.2 Will antimetastatic therapy differ from antiproliferative therapy?

Will antimetastatic therapy be different from antiproliferative therapy [4]? It has been found that the hallmarks of cancer [5] are somewhat different from the hallmarks of metastasis [6]. The hallmarks of cancer are those genes that decide the unlimited growths of cancer cells. However, the hallmarks of metastasis are those genes that decide the interactions between tumor cells and environments (human bodies). They are different types of genes and call for different drugs. However, current clinical chemotherapy mainly provides antiproliferative agents to cancer patients and most patients (90%) die of neoplasm metastasis. One again, let me say that now is the best time to boost our research into more effective antimetastatic drugs [7–8] and apply individualized antimetastatic chemotherapies in clinics [1–2].

5.3 Therapeutic mechanisms of the current antimetastatic drugs

Primary tumors are embedded in a surrounding matrix. Tumor cells and their surrounding matrix can secrete a spectrum of proteinases that will break up this surrounding matrix and make the tumor cells penetrate it, resulting in invasion and metastasis. These proteinases are mainly composed of matrix metalloproteinase (MMPs). So, MMP inhibitors are agents proposed to inhibit tumor metastases. These agents have been licensed since the 1990s in the USA and they are one type of antimetastatic drug [8–10].

Metastatic cells, after extravasation to remote organs, need new blood vessels to offer nutrients to transform the micrometastatic tumor to a macrometastatic nodule. The formation of these blood vessels is controlled by vasculature growth factors, such as EGF, VEGF. Drugs that control the secretion and functions of these vasculature growth factors are known as potential antivascular antimetastatic drugs [11–12].

These two types of antimetastatic drugs are the main source of current antimetastatic therapy in clinics [8].

5.4 Drawbacks of current clinical antimetastatic therapy

Current antimetastatic treatments are overburdened with research into and applications of antivascular (angiogenesis) and matrix metalloproteinase (MMP) inhibitors and more than 500 related agents of different chemical formulae have been reported. Currently most FDA-licensed or internationally available antimetastatic drugs have been categorized as these two types [7–12]. Paradoxically, in view of our efforts and expectations, almost no obvious improvements or therapeutic benefits from conventional antimetastatic drugs (usually antivascular agents or MMP inhibitors) have been achieved. Therapeutic benefits in late-stage or aged cancer patients are especially poor and useless [13–14]. More importantly, some unfavorable side effects of these inhibitors in humans have been reported [15–18]. Also, phase III MMP-inhibitor studies showed that there are no therapeutic benefits of MMP inhibitors for cancer metastasis in terms of patient survival [18]. Clinical antimetastatic drug therapies should change focus to new targets [3]. Both finding important drugs and targeting new antimetastatic pathways are essential and indispensable [3,7–8,19–20]. However, these attempts have not given rise to many new licensed drugs.

5.5 Should human tumor metastasis be treated according to clinical situations —individualized antimetastatic therapy? [19,21–22]

Current antimetastatic therapy treats patients equally. No specific attention is paid in prescribing to the clinical pathological situations of patients.

Tumor metastases involve a fixed course of pathophysiological processes. Human cancer metastasis encompasses several different substages:

1. invade locally through surrounding extracellular matrix (ECM) and stromal cell layers;
2. intravasate into the lumina of blood vessels;
3. tumor cells survive the rigors of transport through the vasculature;
4. arrest at distant organ sites;
5. tumor cells extravasate into the parenchyma of distant tissues;
6. they initially survive in these foreign microenvironments in order to form micrometastases, and
7. reinitiate their proliferative programs at distant sites, thereby generating macroscopic, clinically detectable neoplastic growths [19,23–26].

From this pathological point of view, since a metastasis must travel through more than one body organ, the different anatomic organs may possibly trigger different molecules and pathways linking neoplasm metastases. It follows logically that tumor cells will be affected or inhibited by different types of drugs in different stages of metastatic processes. By the same token, different anticancer drugs will certainly not act in the same way in all metastatic organs [19,21–22].

In general, it was proposed that the MMP inhibitors might be more active in preventing tumor cells from detaching in primary locations [18]. It has been shown that only 1/1,000,000,000 to 1/5,000,000,000 of tumor cells can survive in vascular or lymphatic circulation and finally produce remote forms of metastatic tumor cells [27]. Immuno-modulators might promote the activity of macrophages in killing tumor cells during vascular and lymphatic circulation [28–29]. Thus, immune promoters can inhibit tumor metastasis occurring via tumor-cell blood transportations. On the other hand, tumor cell congregations are less easily targeted by human immune cells. Thus, blood coagulating molecules, such as fibrinogen or thrombin, their biological states can also decide the rate of tumor metastasis [30–36]. Angiogenesis inhibitors might be used at the substage of the attaching of tumor cells to remote organs and micrometastasis formation. However, highly cytotoxic agents might be more effective in the treatment of formed metastatic foci and preference organs [21–22]. See *Figure 5.1.

5.6 Find more metastatis-related molecules and develop novel types of antimetastatic drugs

Current antimetastatic therapies rely heavily on angiogenesis or MMP inhibitors. Since tumor metastasis is a very complex process that triggers more than 100 molecules, other metastatis-related molecules and the development of novel types of antimetastatic drugs are also very important [30–50]. This research needs to be boosted. It might also be very useful in antimetastatic therapy.

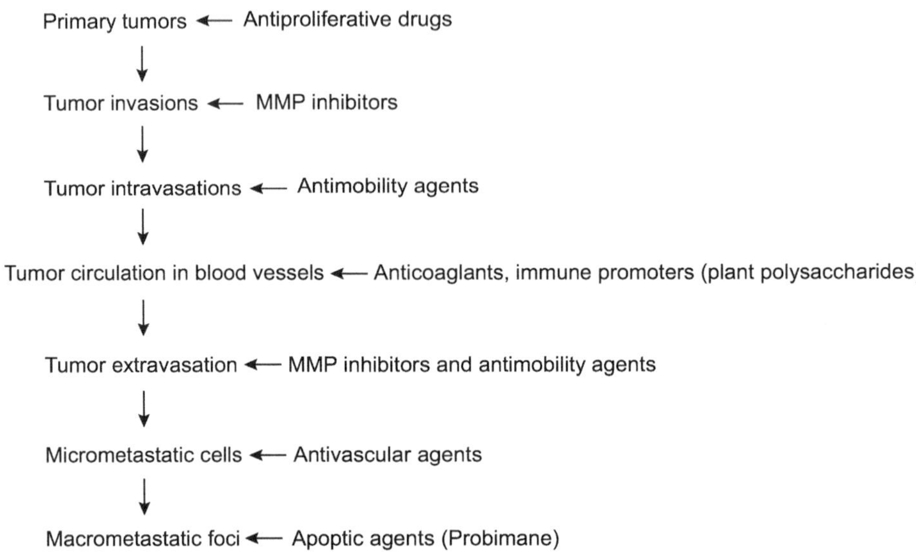

Figure 5.1 Proposed strategy for using antimetastatic agents in clinics.

5.7 Targeting formed metastatic foci in clinics

5.7.1 Background

Most people who die of cancer, die with formed metastatic cancer. In these patients, MMP inhibitors and antivascular agents do not work all the time. Thus, highly active drugs targeting these metastatic tumors need to be developed. Recently, it has been understood that the transmission of a primary tumor to a metastatic tumor in the body is parallel to the transmission of epithelial to mesenchymal [51–52]. This may help to indicate what is mechanistically different between drugs targeting primary tumors and those targeting formed metastatic tumors (Figures 5.2 and 5.3).

The biological pathways in primary tumors and metastatic tumors are opposite. In primary tumor tissue, tumor cells have epithelial-mesenchymal transmission, and in formed metastatic foci, tumor cells have mesenchymal-epithelial transmission, so we propose here that anticancer agents inhibiting primary tumors might be promoters of metastatic tissue. Future strategies for targeting formed metastatic foci need to be boosted.

5.7.2 New strategies targeting formed metastatic foci

In formed metastatic tumor tissues, LY2157299 [19] or probimane [24,54] or apoptotic agents [55] might be more effectively active. Some new types of antimetastatic

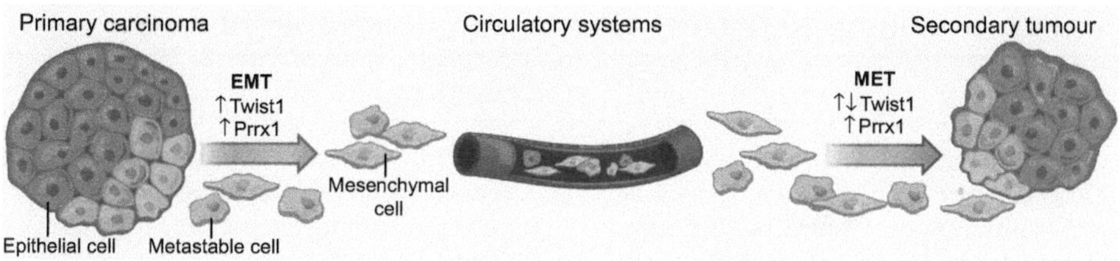

Figure 5.2 Overall picture of primary tumor and metastatic tumors [53].

Primary tumors (EMT) → Blood or lymphatic vessels → Metastatic Foci (MET)

Figure 5.3 Extracting figure of EMT to MET in clinical tumors.

agents, such as agents inhibiting neoplasm sialic acids [37–41] might also be effective against formed metastases. More research is needed.

5.8 Discussion

Individualized antimetastatic therapy studies and clinical utilization still have a long way to go. The paramount task is to find effective drugs to target formed metastases. Presently, the best way of managing antimetastatic drugs targeting formed metastatic foci is to combine cytotoxic anticancer drugs with therapeutic antibodies or other cytostatic anticancer agents [56–62]. But the cost of antibodies is high. The human immune system will produce immune effects in response to these antibodies after several months, owing to the immune defensive mechanisms of the human body [63]. In future, we shall design and develop more effective and less costly antimetastatic drugs, and focused antimetastatic therapy for individuals.

5.9 Conclusion

A decision regarding antimetastatic treatment is best based on the stage of a metastasis in the patient. This would represent a broadening of the current view, where antimetastatic drugs are selected only as a complementary strategy to individualized cancer chemotherapy.

Since tumor metastasis is the main cause of cancer mortality and current clinical therapeutic options are unsatisfactory, more attention must be paid to this research (Table 5.1). Since the population of cancer patients is so large, improvements based on this procedure will save many lives.

Table 5.1 Roadmap to perfect clinical antimetastatic therapy

Methods	Utilizations
New drug target screen	Antimetastatic drug developments
Drug administration or schedule analysis	Treatments with high efficiency
Mechanistic study of antimetastatic drugs	Better use of antimetastatic drugs
Diagnostic studies	Find out if a patient needs antimetastatic drugs
Metastatic cascade study	Proper use of antimetastatic therapy
New active antimetastatic drugs	Formed metastatic foci and tumors

References

[1] D.Y. Lu, T.R. Lu, X.L. Chen, J. Ding, Individualized Cancer Chemotherapy, in: M.M. Shoja, P.S. Agutter, R.S. Tubbs, M. Ghanei, K. Ghabili et al. (Eds.), Hypotheses in Clinical Medicine, Nova Science Publishers, Hauppage, NY, 2012. chapter 13.
[2] D.Y. Lu, T.R. Lu, H.Y. Wu, New insights into individualized antimetastatic therapy, Adv. Tech. Biol. Med. 1 (1) (2013) 106.
[3] D.Y. Lu, T.R. Lu, Antimetastatic activities and mechanisms of bisdioxopiperazine compounds, Anti-Canc. Agent. Med. Chem. 10 (7) (2010) 564–570.
[4] L.A. Mina, G.W. Sledge, Rethinking the metastatic cascade as a therapeutic target, Nature Rev. Clin. Oncol. 8 (2011) 325–332.
[5] D. Hanahan, R.A. Weinberg, The hallmarks of cancer, Cell 100 (1) (2000) 57–70.
[6] G.P. Gupta, J. Massagué, Cancer metastasis: building a framework, Cell 127 (2006) 679–695.
[7] D.Y. Lu, T.R. Lu, S. Cao, Cancer metastases and clinical therapies, Cell Develop. Biol. 1 (4) (2012) e110.
[8] D.Y. Lu, T.R. Lu, H.Y. Wu, S. Cao, Cancer metastases treatments, Curr. Drug Ther. 8 (1) (2013) 24–29.
[9] G. Sava, A. Bergamo, Drug control of solid tumour metastases: a critical view, Anticancer Res. 19 (2A) (1999) 1117–1124.
[10] K. Kessenbrock, V. Plaks, Z. Werb, Matrix metalloproteinases: regulators of the tumor microenvironment, Cell 141 (1) (2010) 52–67.
[11] G. Taraboletti, B. Margosio, Antiangiogenic and antivascular therapy for cancer, Curr. Opin. Pharmacol. 1 (4) (2001) 378–384.
[12] J. Folkman, Angiogenesis, Ann. Rev. Med. 57 (2006) 1–18.
[13] H. Varmus, The new era in cancer research, Science 312 (5777) (2006) 1162–1165.
[14] A. Jemal, et al., Cancer statistics 2006, CA, Cancer J. Clin. 56 (2) (2006) 106–130.
[15] M. Paez-Ribes, et al., Antiangiogenic therapy elicits malignant progression of tumors to increased local invasion and distant metastasis, Cancer Cell 15 (3) (2009) 220–231.
[16] J.M.L. Ebos, et al., Accelerated metastasis after short-term treatment with a potent inhibitor of tumor angiogenesis, Cancer Cell 15 (3) (2009) 232–239.
[17] H.M. Verheul, H.M. Pinedo, Possible molecular mechanisms involved in the toxicity of angiogenesis inhibition, Nature Rev. Cancer 7 (6) (2007) 475–485.
[18] L.M. Coussens, B. Fingleton, L.M. Matrisian, Matrix metalloproteinase inhibitors and cancer: trials and tribulations, Science 295 (2002) 2387–2392.

[19] S. Valastyan, R.A. Weinberg, Tumor metastasis: molecular insights and evolving paradigms, Cell 147 (2) (2011) 275–292.

[20] F. Dong, A.S. Budhu, X.W. Wang, Translating the metastasis paradigm from scientific theory to clinical oncology, Clin. Cancer Res. 15 (8) (2009) 2588–2593.

[21] D.Y. Lu, F.G. Wu, Z.M. Shen, T.R. Lu, H.Y. Wu, et al., Different spontaneous pulmonary metastasis inhibitions against lewis lung carcinoma in mice by bisdioxopiperazine compounds of different treatment schedules, Scientia Pharm. 78 (2010) 13–20.

[22] D.Y. Lu, Y.C. Xi, Antimetastatic therapies according to metastatic cascade, Adv. Pharma. Drug Safety 1 (2012) e107.

[23] G. Poste, I.J. Fidler, The pathogenesis of cancer metastasis, Nature 283 (5743) (1980) 139–146.

[24] I.J. Fidler, Critical factors in the biology of human cancer metastasis. Twenty-eighth G H A clowes memorial awards lecture, Cancer Res. 50 (19) (1990) 6130–6138.

[25] I.J. Fidler, The pathogenesis of cancer metastasis: the 'seed and soil' hypothesis revisited, Nature Rev. Cancer 3 (6) (2003) 453–458.

[26] C.A. Klein, The metastasis cascade, Science 321 (5897) (2008) 1785–1787.

[27] V. Marx, Tracking metastasis and tricking cancer, Nature 494 (2013) 133–138.

[28] I.J. Fidler, Macrophages and metastasis—A biological approach to cancer therapy: Presidential address, Cancer Res. 45 (1985) 4714–4726.

[29] M. Cristofanilli, G. Thomas Budd, Matthew J. Ellis, Alison Stopeck, Jeri Matera, et al., Circulating tumor cells, disease progression, and survival in metastatic breast cancer, N. Engl. J. Med. 351 (2004) 781–791.

[30] D.Y. Lu, J.Y. Cao, Y.P. Huang, L. Gong, X.L. Chen, et al., Comparison of some antineoplastic drugs on inhibiting thrombin catalyzing fibrinogen clotting in vitro, Chin. Med. J. (Eng.) 112 (11) (1999) 1052–1053.

[31] D.Y. Lu, X.L. Chen, J.Y. Cao, Z. Li, H.W. Xue, et al., Effects of cancer chemotherapy on the blood fibrinogen concentrations of cancer patients, J. Int. Med. Res. 28 (6) (2000) 313–317, 2000.

[32] D.Y. Lu, J. Chi, L.P. Lin, M. Huang, B. Xu, et al., Effect of anti-cancer drugs on the binding of ^{125}I-Fibrinogen to two leukemia cell lines in vitro, Int. J. Med. Res. 32 (5) (2004) 488–491.

[33] D.Y. Lu, Inhibiting the synthesis and functions of fibrinogen in tumors with normal anticancer drugs, a novel target for cancer chemotherapy, 96th Ann. Meeting Proc. AACR 46 (2005) 1396–1397.

[34] D.Y. Lu, X.L. Chen, J. Ding, Treatment of solid tumors and metastases by fibrinogen-targeted anticancer drug therapy, Med. Hypotheses 68 (1) (2007) 188–193.

[35] V. Bobek, Anticoagulant and fibrinolytic drugs—possible agents in treatment of lung cancer? Anticancer Agent Med. Chem. 12 (6) (2012) 580–588.

[36] P. Rothwell, F.G. Fowkes, J.F. Belch, H. Ogawa, C.P. Warlow, et al., Effect of daily aspirin on long-term risk of death due to cancer: analysis of individual patient data from randomized trials, Lancet 377 (2011) 31–41.

[37] D.Y. Lu, J.Y. Cao, Structural aberration of cellular sialic acids and their functions in cancer, J. Shanghai Univ. (Eng.) 5 (2) (2001) 164–170.

[38] D.Y. Lu, T.R. Lu, H.Y. Wu, Antimetastatic therapy targeting aberrant sialylation profiles in cancer cells, Drugs Ther. Stud. 1 (1) (2011) e12.

[39] D.Y. Lu, T.R. Lu, H.Y. Wu, Development of antimetastatic drugs by targeting tumor sialic acids, Scientia Pharm. 80 (3) (2012) 497–508.

[40] Y.C. Xi, D.Y. Lu, Relationship between tumor sialic acids and neoplasm metastasis and as a drug target, Cell Dev. Biol. 1 (2012) e106.

[41] D.Y. Lu, J. Xu, T.R. Lu, H.Y. Wu, B. Xu, Inhibitions of several antineoplastic drugs on serum sialic acid levels in mice bearing tumors, Scientia Pharm. 81 (1) (2013) 223–231.

[42] V. Vetvicka, M. Fusek, Procathepsin D as a tumor marker, anti-cancer drug or screening agent, Anticancer Agent Med. Chem. 12 (2) (2012) 172–175.
[43] L. Chen, S. Yang, J. Jakoncic, J.J. Zhang, X.Y. Huang, Migrastatin analogues target fascin to block tumor metastasis, Nature 464 (7291) (2010) 1062–1066.
[44] S. Valastyan, F. Reinhardt, N. Benaich, D. Calogrias, A. Szasz, et al., A pleiotropically acting microRNA, miR-31, inhibits breast cancer metastasis, Cell 137 (6) (2009) 1032–1046.
[45] G.F. Nash, L.F. Turner, M.F. Scully, A.K. Kakkar, Platelets and cancer, Lancet Oncol. 3 (7) (2002) 425–430.
[46] M. Iiizumi, W. Liu, S.K. Pai, E. Furuta, K. Watabe, Drug development against metastasis-related genes and pathways: a rationale for cancer therapy, BBA 1786 (2) (2008) 87–104.
[47] D.Y. Lu, T.R. Lu, J. Ding, Cell biological manifestations of bisdioxopiperazines: treatment of human tumor cell lines in culture, Anticancer Agent Med. Chem. 10 (9) (2010) 657–660.
[48] S.L. Goodman, M. Picard, Integrins as therapeutic targets, Trends Pharm. Sci. 33 (7) (2012) 405–412.
[49] J. Paredes, J. Figueiredo, A. Albergaria, P. Oliveira, J. Carvalho, et al., Epithelial E- and P-cadherins, role and clinical significance in cancer, BBA 1826 (2) (2012) 297–311.
[50] G. Bendas, L. Borsig, Cancer cell adhesion and metastasis, selectins, integrins, and the inhibitory potential of heparins, Int. J. Cell Biol. (2012) 676731.
[51] J.P. Thiery, H. Acloque, R.Y. Huang, M.A. Nieto, Epithelial-mesenchymal transitions in development and disease, Cell 139 (5) (2009) 871–890.
[52] R. Kalluri, R.A. Weinberg, The basics of epithelial-mesenchymal transition, J. Clin. Invest. 119 (6) (2009) 1420–1428.
[53] B.J.W. Van Denderen, E.W. Thompson, Cancer: the to and fro of tumour spread, Nature 493 (2013) 487–488.
[54] D.Y. Lu, T.R. Lu, Anticancer activities and mechanisms of bisdioxopiperazine compounds probimane and MST-16, Anticancer Agent Med. Chem. 10 (1) (2010) 78–91.
[55] P. Mehlen, A. Puisieux, Metastasis; a question of life or death, Nature Rev. Cancer 6 (6) (2006) 449–458.
[56] D.Y. Lu, T.R. Lu, H.Y. Wu, Combination chemical agents with biological means in cancer therapy, Res. Rev. BioSci. 7 (4) (2013) 153–155.
[57] R.J. Lechleider, E. Kaminskas, X. Jiang, R. Aziz, J. Bullock, R. Kasliwal, et al., Ixabepilone in combination with capecitabine and as monotherapy for treatment of advanced breast cancer refractory to previous chemotherapies, Clin. Cancer Res. 14 (14) (2008) 4378–4384.
[58] D.L. Gillespie, K. Whang, B.T. Ragel, J.R. Flynn, D.A. Kelly, et al., Silencing of hypoxia inducible factor-1α by RNA interference attenuates human glioma cell growth in vivo, Clin. Cancer Res. 13 (2007) 2441–2448.
[59] C.E. Geyer, et al., Lapatinib plus capecitabine for HER2-positive advanced breast cancer, N. Engl. J. Med. 355 (2006) 2733–2743.
[60] J.B. Vermorken, R. Mesia, F. Rivera, E. Remenar, A. Kawecki, et al., Platinum-based chemotherapy plus cetuximab in head and neck cancer, N. Engl. J. Med. 359 (2008) 1116–1127.
[61] A. Younes, N.L. Bartlett, J.P. Leonard, D.A. Kennedy, C.M. Lynch, et al., Brentuximab vedotin (SGN-35) for relapsed CD30-positive lymphomas, N. Engl. J. Med. 363 (2010) 1812–1821.
[62] The Lancet Oncology, New hope for advanced gastric cancer, Lancet Oncol. 11 (3) (2010) 211.
[63] C. Warnke, C. Hermanrud, M. Lundkvist, A. Fogdell-Hahn, Anti-drug antibodies, Drugs Ther. Stud. 2 (1) (2012) e11.

Drug combinations

6

6.1 Introduction

Most cancers have multiple genetic alterations or abnormalities. Only one anticancer drug is seldom adequate [1–2]. Human cancer is a refractory and resistant disease, and like the HIV virus, it might call for a drug cocktail rather than a single drug to control the progress of the disease effectively [3–8]. A drug cocktail may be one of the good solutions in anticancer chemotherapy. How to combine anticancer drugs in practice is a new problem and area in anticancer drug therapy. Most cancers have multiple genetic alterations and molecular abnormalities. It is seldom very useful by using only one anticancer drug owing to refractory and drug resistance of cancer tissues. Anticancer drug cocktail instead single drugs might dramatically promote the control of cancer progresses and metastasis in different patients. Despite it becomes a modern cliché that anticancer drug combination is better than single anticancer drug, how to combinative utilizations of anticancer drug cocktails is a new series of problems and solutions in new era of anticancer therapy studies. Most important, anticancer drug cocktails need transformation from empirical to science-guided systems. This chapter pictures the scenarios and landscapes of present and future knowledge of cancer therapy, especially possible future solutions for overcoming weaknesses, limitations, pitfalls and drawbacks of past cancer therapy and create more matured ones.

6.2 Cytotoxic drugs and biotherapy

6.2.1 *Background*

Cancer is a high-mortality disease and the therapeutics for cancer, especially for cancer metastasis, is still imperfect. Many cancer patients die of metastases [9–12]. One of the reasons for the unsatisfactory state of cancer therapy is the toxicity of antineoplastic drugs to human bodies. Anticancer drugs can be divided into two categories—cytotoxic anticancer drugs and cytostatic anticancer drugs [13]. Cytotoxic antineoplastic drugs are very toxic and will kill normal human cells at the same time as cancer cells. So dosages of antineoplastic drugs in therapy must not be too high, or patients cannot tolerate them. In the end, a small proportion of cancer cells survives after cytotoxic anticancer drug chemotherapy. These tumor cells will regrow to become large tumors and multidrug resistance (MDR) often occurs in these cells. It is these cancer cells or metastatic cancer cells that kill patients. The best method is to combine cytotoxic anticancer chemicals with cytostatic anticancer drugs, antimetastatic drugs or biotherapies (Table 6.1).

The best strategy in anticancer therapy is to effectuate and update the present therapeutic norm. One method being attempted is to combine cytotoxic chemicals and

Personalized Cancer Chemotherapy.

Table 6.1 Different anticancer biotherapies

Biotherapy	Targets
Monoclonal or polyclonal antibodies	Tumor biomarkers
Vaccines	Tumor antigens
Gene therapy	Escalated tumor genes or antigens
Cytokine therapy	Human tumor environment
Immune therapy	Tumor antigen
iRNA	Tumor genes

biotherapies. If cytotoxic anticancer chemical drugs can kill 70% to 95% of tumor cells, some highly specific biotherapies will kill the rest of the tumor cells with no obvious toxicities [7–8]. This is our ultimate goal. This strategy is a paradigm of future cancer chemotherapy. It is well known that anticancer drugs rarely kill all tumor cells. If several cancer cells remain, they will quickly regrow to produce a large cancer. So immuno-surveillance systems for patients or the effects of highly specific biotherapies [8] will decide long-term effectiveness for patients. The development of biotherapies that are currently insufficient will be the great task of future therapeutic studies. The best paradigm in use today is to combine cytotoxic anticancer chemicals with monoclonal or polyclonal antibodies [7–8,14–23]. On the other hand, other biological means, such as vaccines, can also combine with cytotoxic chemotherapy.

6.3 The advantages of a strategy of combining cytotoxic anticancer drugs and biotherapy

Biotherapies for cancer are often relatively mild and very costly and ineffective against large-volume tumors. Yet they are highly specific and kill only a few tumor cells with completeness and no toxicity. Cytotoxic anticancer chemotherapy should always be given before a specific biotherapy. The job of the cytotoxic chemical drugs is to reduce the tumor to a minimum volume, then highly specific biotherapy will kill the rest of the tumor cells, no matter whether these tumor cells are MDR or not. This is a perfect strategy and should be the way to achieve a better outcome [7–8].

6.3.1 Challenge for this strategy

The strategy outlined above is a perfect strategy and anticancer drug combination [7–8]. But some problems and challenges remain.

- First, current biotherapy is not perfect. The cytotoxicity of most current biotherapy is weak, and will seldom completely destroy all cancer cells if the tumor volume is more than 0.5 cm. We need to innovate and produce more effective biotherapy for cancer, especially against formed metastatic foci, because these are the main cause of cancer patients' deaths.

- Secondly, we do not know which biological pathways go aberrant in specific tumors in clinics. We must first know the characteristics of the tumor to be treated by detecting tumor biomarkers or bioinformatics [5,7]. Then we can design suitable biotherapy regimes.
- The third reason is the high cost of biotherapy, especially antibody and microRNA. So a patient's financial status is an important factor in deciding whether we can use biotherapy or not. On the other hand, therapeutic antibodies inhibit cancer growth or metastasis for only a few months. After the administration of therapeutic antibodies for several months, a human body will produce an immune response against therapeutic antibodies [24]. Then the therapeutic effects of antibodies will be terminated.

There is a long way to go and more effort is required of us. The more we focus our attention on this matter, the more satisfactory the results we can anticipate.

6.4 Combined use of both antiproliferative drugs (primary tumor) and antimetastatic drugs

Apart from manufacturing more effective and specific anticancer or antimetastatic drugs, combined use of antiproliferative drugs (primary tumor) and antimetastatic drugs is a sound strategy to prolong survival. The proper use of antimetastatic drugs was discussed in chapter 5.

6.5 Combined cytotoxic drugs and cytostatic drugs

The combined use of cytostatic and cytotoxicity anticancer drugs must be based on detection of cancer biomarkers. Anticancer drugs are divided into two categories; cytotoxic and cytostatic drugs. Cytotoxic drugs indiscriminately kill cancer and normal tissue. They are effective on almost all types of cancer cells, but also often toxic to normal tissue, and very easily provoke multi-drug resistance (MDR). So cytotoxic anticancer drugs cannot be used in very high doses or for long enough to kill all cancer cells.

Cytostatic anticancer drugs target specific mutated genes, molecules or receptors. Though the overall antiproliferative effects of cytostatic anticancer drugs are lower than those of cytotoxic anticancer drugs, they are much less toxic to normal tissue and their tumor responses are relatively long-lasting.

The use of cytostatic anticancer drugs, selected according to the abnormality of tumor markers in individual patients, is a selective and evaluated system. Each important abnormality in cancer markers will be targeted by relevant cytostatic drugs [5]. By using the combination of cytotoxic anticancer drugs with cytostatic anticancer drugs, we can render the drug response to tumors very high or can even eradicate tumors. This type of drug combination might be chosen based on the detection of tumor markers or cancer bioinformatics.

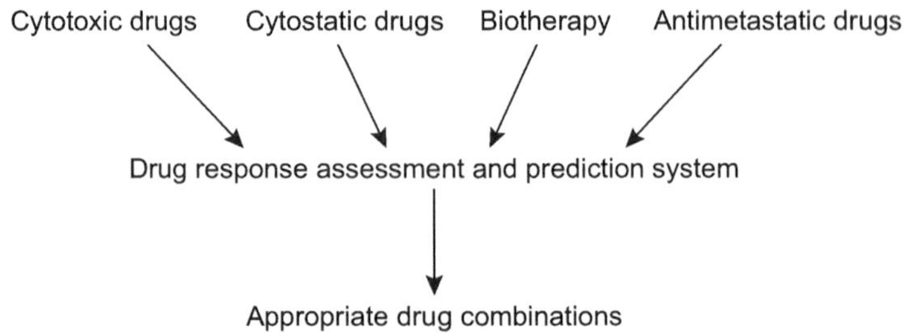

Figure 6.1 The general protocols of drug combinations.

6.6 Rules of drug combination

As with an HIV cocktail, the best drug combination is of drugs targeting different mechanisms (Figure 6.1). The more diversified the drug types, the more integrated benefits a therapy might have. However, if we can find out the drug-sensitivity test results of cytotoxic anticancer drugs and the drug response of cytostatic anticancer drugs on a specific tumor species by detecting cancer biomarkers, may we have a better therapeutic outcome?

6.7 Conclusion

Generally speaking, a drug combination has better therapeutic outcomes than single anticancer drug treatment. But concomitantly, it often costs much more than a single drug. The consideration of cost-effectiveness for drug combinations is one part of the work of a clinician and in basic cancer chemotherapy studies, especially when costly drugs are proposed.

Mounting experimental data and clinical evidence suggest it might be optimal to use drug combinations in controlling tumor growth and metastasis. However, the toxicities of drug combinations to humans are increased with the increase of drug numbers. Drug sensitivity tests, cancer biomarker detection and pharmacogenetics are designed to select effective drugs and to discard ineffective drugs. They can effect a good balance between drug activity and toxicity.

References

[1] P.C. Nowell, The clonal evolution of tumor cell populations, Sci. 194 (4260) (1976) 23–28 (Washington DC).
[2] D. Hanahan, R.A. Weinberg, The hallmarks of cancer, Cell 100 (1) (2000) 57–70.
[3] A.J. Tipping, J.V. Melo, Imatinib mesylate in combination with other chemotherapeutic drugs: in vitro studies, Semin Hematol. 40 (2) (2003) 83–91.
[4] B. Druker, Imatinib alone and in combination for chronic myeloid leukemia, Semin Hematol. 40 (1) (2003) 50–58.
[5] A. Ocaña, A. Pandiella, Personalized therapies in the cancer "omics" era, Mol. Cancer 9 (2010) 202.

[6] R.L. Strausberg, A.J. Simpson, L.J. Old, G.J. Riggins, Oncogenomics and the development of new cancer therapies, Nature 429 (6990) (2004) 469–474 2004.
[7] D.Y. Lu, T.R. Lu, X.L. Chen, J. Ding, Individualized cancer chemotherapy, in: M.M. Shoja, P.S. Agutter, R.S. Tubbs, M. Ghanei, K. Ghabili et al. (Eds.), Hypotheses in Clinical Medicine, Nova Science Publishers, Hauppage, NY, 2012, pp. 199–216. chapter 13.
[8] D.Y. Lu, T.R. Lu, H.Y. Wu, Combination chemical agents with biological means in cancer therapy, Res. Rev. BioSci. 7 (4) (2013) 153–155.
[9] D.Y. Lu, T.R. Lu, S. Cao, Cancer metastases and clinical therapies, Cell Dev. Biol. 1 (2012) e110.
[10] S. Valastyan, R.A. Weinberg, Tumor metastasis: molecular insights and evolving paradigms, Cell 147 (2) (2011) 275–292.
[11] D.Y. Lu, T.R. Lu, H.Y. Wu, New insights into individualized antimetastatic therapy, Adv. Tech. Biol. Med. 1 (2013) 106.
[12] D.Y. Lu, T.R. Lu, H.Y. Wu, S. Cao, Cancer metastases treatments, Curr. Drug Ther. 8 (1) (2013) 24–29.
[13] A.W. Millar, K.P. Lynch, Rethinking clinical trials for cytostatic drugs, Nature Rev. Cancer 3 (7) (2003) 540–545.
[14] R.J. Lechleider, E. Kaminskas, X. Jiang, R. Aziz, J. Bullock, R. Kasliwal, et al., Ixabepilone in combination with capecitabine and as monotherapy for treatment of advanced breast cancer refractory to previous chemotherapies, Clin. Cancer Res. 14 (14) (2008) 4378–4384.
[15] D.L. Gillespie, K. Whang, B. T. Ragel, J.R. Flynn, D.A. Kelly, et al., Silencing of hypoxia inducible factor-1α by RNA interference attenuates human glioma cell growth *In vivo*, Clin. Cancer Res. 13 (2007) 2441–2448.
[16] C.E. Geyer, et al., Lapatinib plus capecitabine for HER2-positive advanced breast cancer, N. Engl. J. Med. 355 (2006) 2733–2743.
[17] J.B. Vermorken, et al., Platinum-based chemotherapy plus cetuximab in head and neck cancer, N. Engl. J. Med. 359 (2008) 1116–1127.
[18] A. Younes, N.L. Bartlett, J.P. Leonard, D.A. Kennedy, C.M. Lynch, et al., Brentuximab vedotin (SGN-35) for relapsed CD30-positive lymphomas, N. Engl. J. Med. 363 (2010) 1812–1821.
[19] The Lancet Oncology, New hope for advanced gastric cancer, Lancet Oncol. 11 (3) (2010) 211.
[20] K. Miller, M. Wang, J. Gralow, et al., Paclitaxel plus bevacizumab versus paclitaxel alone for metastatic breast cancer, N. Engl. J. Med. 357 (2007) 2666–2676.
[21] J. Tol, M. Koopman, A. Cats, et al., Chemotherapy, bevacizumab, and cetuximab in metastatic colorectal cancer, N. Engl. J. Med. 360 (2009) 563–572.
[22] E.D. Ball, H.E. Broom, Monoclonal antibodies in the treatment of hematologic malignancy, Best Pract. Res. Clin. Haematol. 23 (3) (2010) 403–416.
[23] A. Naeim, E.B. Keeler, Is adjuvant therapy for older patients with node (-) early breast cancer cost-effective? Crit. Rev. Oncol. Hematol. 53 (1) (2005) 81–89.
[24] C. Warnke, C. Hermanrud, M. Lundkvist, A. Fogdell-Hahn, Anti-drug antibodies, Drugs Ther. Stud. 2 (1) (2012) e11.

Assistant chemotherapy

7

Causes of death for cancer patients in clinics can be multi-factorial. Apart from the direct causes of tumor progression and metastases, other clinical complications or psychiatric factors will hasten death. It is known that certain assistant therapies can be harmful to cancer patients who have clinical complications or psychiatric problems [1]. On the other hand, many recent findings have shown that assistant therapies will ameliorate fatal symptoms and prolong patients' survival. Further research is required in this area. Assistant cancer therapy was a long originated clinical practice for cancer patients. Many of them have been speculated for more than half century, such as anti-venous thrombosis therapy for solid human tumors and traditional Chinese medicine. In order to promote these kinds of researches and clinical trials, systematic creative investigations are needed and renewed. Many clinical knowhow also play key role for these reaches.

7.1 Anti-thrombosis therapy

7.1.1 History and examples

Next to cancer metastasis, the second deadly pathological feature of cancer patients is venous thromboembolism [2]. Venous thromboembolism has caused numerous cancer deaths. Assistant therapies that have been proposed include the use of anticoagulants and / or fibrinolytic agents such as warfarin, heparin, and oxalysine.

Disordered coagulation is encountered in up to 90% of cancer patients with solid tumors, and 15% of them develop a localized acute or chronic deep thrombosis. The causes of disordered coagulation can be multifactorial events, such as neoplasm metastasis, chemotherapy or hormone therapy (impairing the blood vessel walls or promoting a coagulation cascade), venous catheters, both in use and immobilized [2]. Disordered coagulation can also be caused by multiple blood components, platelets [3], plasma and the tumor matrix of fibrinogen [4–17] and coagulant components, such as thrombin [6–10]. Most importantly, cancer patients with venous thromboembolism symptoms have been considered for assistant therapy of anticoagulants and / or fibrinolytic agents such as warfarin, heparin, tissue plasminogen activator or oxalysine [1–17] for prolonging survival.

7.1.2 Prevention in surgical patients

Cancer patients who undergo surgery are at high risk of developing a thromboembolic complication. They have twice the risk of postoperative deep venous thrombosis (DVT) and more than three times the risk of a fatal pulmonary embolism than patients who undergo surgery for benign disease. Now, there is a consensus that prophylactic low-doses of heparin (5000 IU daily for 8 to 12 hours starting 1 to 2 hours before the

Personalized Cancer Chemotherapy.

operation) should be used in patients undergoing malignant tissue surgery. A subgroup analysis of cancer patients revealed that low-dose unfractioned heparin is able to reduce DVT from 22% (control) to 9% in cancer patients.

Only in non-surgery cancer patients, prophylactic antithrombosis therapy can be used with a central venous catheter, because central venous catheters will increase the incidence of deep venous thrombosis (DVT) and death.

7.1.3 Choice among different drugs

Anticoagulants and / or fibrinolytic agents are many, including warfarin, low-molecular-weight heparin, unfractionated heparin, tissue plasminogen activators, urikonase and clicumarol. Among these anticoagulants and / or fibrinolytic agents, warfarin and low-molecular-weight heparin (LMWH) are especially used in clinics. Warfarin is given orally, and it seems to be easily handled. However, there is a great risk of bleeding (haemorrhagic complications) or ineffectiveness in cancer patients who take warfarin because of inappropriate blood or plasma concentrations of warfarin in patients' bodies. This is because there is great variation in the bioavailability of warfarin in human bodies. The bioavailability of warfarin can be affected by many drugs that interfere with the synthesis of hepatic cytochrome P450 (CYP metabolizing enzymes). The bioavailability of warfarin is affected by the polymorphism of CYP-metabolizing enzymes. So caution is essential when other drugs are used with warfarin. Further, warfarin can prolong 5-fluorouracil half-life via its potential interaction with other drugs [16]. Thus precise control of the dosage of warfarin in cancer patients is very difficult. There are two possible solutions for this problem. One is to constantly monitor patients' blood-coagulate status (correct INR level is between 1.3 and 1.9). This is a very cumbersome task. The second way is to use pharmacogenomics in deciding warfarin doses. But low-molecular-weight heparin (LMWH) or unfractionated heparin, is intravenously or subcutaneously administered and easy to handle. Many patients who fail in warfarin therapy are improved by LMWH or other intravenously injected drugs. Dalteparin (200 IU/Kg daily for 5-7 days) can be administered subcutaneously. It is easier to handle.

7.1.4 Cancer categories targeted by anti-thrombosis therapy

The other important issue is to know which categories of solid cancer are suitable for prophylactic anti-thrombosis therapy. In most cases, anti-thrombosis therapy does not significantly improve survival rates. Only 1/3 of cancer patients benefited from this therapy [7]. However, survival rates have been greatly improved in patients with lung cancer, especially non-small-cell lung cancer, with anti-thrombosis therapy [12]. Survival rates are also improved anti-thrombosis therapy in patients with breast cancer [2]. Overall, patients with solid tumors are likely to improve with the use of anticoagulant or fibrinolytic agent therapies [10].

7.1.5 Anti-thrombosis therapy combined with anticancer drugs

Anti-thrombosis therapy is an assistant therapy. Success is seldom achieved with anticoagulants alone. Common anticancer drugs are the mainstay of these therapies and they are active to a greater or lesser extent on the body's coagulate system. Conventional first-line anticancer drugs can affect the binding of fibrinogen with tumor cells [9,14] and at the same time contribute to blood coagulation changes (up or down) in cancer patients [2–3]. If we combine anticancer drugs with anti-coagulants, we can expect cooperative effects between them. Thus anti-thrombosis therapy must be combined with anticancer drugs. With this combined treatment, a reduced risk of developing liver metastasis has been reported in fluorouracil / heparin groups, compared to surgery alone or intraportal infusion of urikonase for 24 hours ($P<0.01$) alone. No advantage was reported in the group treated with heparin alone [16].

7.1.6 Conclusion

Anticoagulants and/or fibrinolytic agents as an assistant therapy for solid cancers can obviously prolong patients' survival, especially in lung cancer, and are a promising strategy in cancer therapy, especially in the treatment of cancer metastases and thrombosis-related deaths. However, some meta-analysis reports have showed that many types of solid tumor have been improved very little with the use of heparin in clinics. It is possible that only small proportions of patients with solid tumors are helped in this way [17]. Previously, anticoagulant prophylaxis in operative ovarian cancer patients has been proved to be cost-effective [18]. So this type of therapy should be more widely used for patients with solid tumors.

7.2 Antidepressant therapy

7.2.1 Utilization of antidepressants in cancer patients

A lot of people believe cancer is an incurable disease. Some of them are terrified after hearing they have contracted cancer. Their mental strength begins to collapse. We all know that the fear of death in cancer patients will speed up the patients' death. It has been hypothesized whether antidepressants can be used as an assistant therapy for patients with psychiatric difficulties. If this type of assistant therapy can ease patients' panic, longer survival periods can be expected [19]. But these therapies are only assistant therapies. They do not target tumor cells, because tumor cells are caused by a genetic abnormality of common cells [20]. Mostly, humans' psychological status is decided by their inherent genetic makeup. Thus, pharmacogenomics studies of patients' inherent genetic makeup will be helpful for determining if antidepressants are needed.

7.2.2 The side effects of antidepressants

Antidepressant may have side effects, including suicide attempts [21]. We have hypothesized that they are linked with patients' genetic status [22–25]. Thus, we conclude that psychological assistant therapy is a complicated enterprise and needs to be studied very carefully.

7.2.3 Conclusion

Utilization of antidepressants in cancer patients is not a very new proposition. But it is seldom attempted in clinics. This may be owing to a lack of successful experimental or clinical outcomes. Also, antidepressants can decrease the efficacy of tamoxifen therapy. In future, let us explore this strategy further.

7.3 Improving patients' physiological conditions

We all know that cancer is a wasting disease and anticancer or antimetastatic drugs are very toxic agents which weaken patients and cause some deaths. Many existing methods are suitable for targeting this situation and looking at its drawbacks.

7.3.1 Traditional Chinese medicine (TCM)

TCM aims to tune up patients' physiological condition and make them stronger and ameliorate physiological problems. TCM is a paradigm of individual therapy. Experienced TCM doctors survey patients' physiological conditions and remedy them, after understanding the underlying deficiencies. These treatments rely on establishing and maintaining a balance between active ('yang') and passive ('yin') energies in different organs and physiological systems [26]. It is a subtle topic which needs many years of experience and comparative data between TCM and Western medicine.

Treatment of cancer by TCM is a hot topic in modern China. There are many favorable reports on TCM in the treatment of cancer patients [27–30].

According to traditional Chinese medicine (TCM), human bodies are formed and balanced by fighting between inner upright strength (正气) and outside damaging air (邪气). Individualized TCM therapy should be based on either strengthening the inner upright energy (补正气) or preventing or expelling the outside damaging air (去邪气). In most cancer cases, according to TCM, patients need to strengthen upright energy and such a therapy might be more beneficial than preventing or expelling outside damaging air. Many TCM doctors in China hold this view.

7.3.2 Assistant treatment with Western drugs

Cancer is a deteriorating and wasting disease. Cancer patients, especially late-stage cancer patients, need more nutrients to keep the body in normal form. This type of assistant therapy, with the use of supplements such as antioxidants or selenium, can be used and is discussed in the works referenced [31–33].

7.4 Conclusion

As assistant treatment for cancer patients, more and more assistant anticancer therapies have been proved to prolong patients' survival. In future, more attention and effort will be focused on these types of assistant treatment. In most cases, assistant therapies needs to be combined with the use of anticancer or antimetastatic drugs, otherwise their therapeutic benefits will be undermined.

References

[1] D.Y. Lu, T.R. Lu, X.L. Chen, J. Ding, Individualized cancer chemotherapy, in: M.M. Shoja, P.S. Agutter, R.S. Tubbs, M. Ghanei, K. Ghabili et al. (Eds.), Hypotheses in Clinical Medicine, Nova Science Publishers, Hauppage, NY, 2012, pp. 199–216. chapter 13.
[2] M. Mandalà, G. Ferretti, M. Cremonesi, M. Cazzaniga, G. Curigliano, et al, Venous thromboembolism and cancer: new issues for an old topic, Crit. Rev. Oncol. Hematol. 48 (1) (2003) 65–80.
[3] G.F. Nash, L.F. Turner, M.F. Scully, A.K. Kakkar, Platelets and cancer, Lancet Oncol. 3 (7) (2002) 425–430.
[4] D.Y. Lu, X.L. Chen, M. Huang, B. Xu, J. Ding, Relationship between blood fibrinogen concentration and pathological features of cancer patients: a 139-case clinical study, OnLine J. Biol. Sci. 7 (1) (2007) 8–11.
[5] D.Y. Lu, X.L. Chen, J.Y. Cao, Z. Li, H.W. Xue, et al., Effects of cancer chemotherapy on the blood fibrinogen concentrations of cancer patients, J. Int. Med. Res. 28 (6) (2000) 313–317.
[6] H.F. Dvorak, D.R. Senger, A.M. Dvorak, Fibrin as a component of the tumor stroma: origins and biological significance, Cancer Metastasis Rev. 2 (1) (1983) 41–73.
[7] V. Costantini, L.R. Zacharski, The role of fibrin in tumor metastasis, Cancer Metastasis Rev. 11 (3–4) (1992) 283–290.
[8] C.A. Staton, N.J. Brown, C.E. Lewis, The role of fibrinogen and related fragments in tumour angiogenesis and metastasis, Expert. Opin. Biol. Ther. 3 (7) (2003) 1105–1120.
[9] D.Y. Lu, J. Chi, L.P. Lin, M. Huang, B. Xu, et al., Effect of anticancer drugs on the binding of ^{125}I-fibrinogen to two leukemia cell lines in vitro, J. Int. Med. Res. 32 (5) (2004) 488–491.
[10] D.Y. Lu, X.L. Chen, J. Ding, Treatment of solid tumors and metastases by fibrinogen-targeted anticancer drug therapy, Med. Hypotheses 68 (1) (2007) 188–193.
[11] D.Y. Lu, J.Y. Cao, Y.P. Huang, L. Gong, X.L. Chen, et al., Comparison of some antineoplastic drugs on inhibiting thrombin catalyzing fibrinogen clotting in vitro, Chin. Med. J. (Eng.) 112 (11) (1999) 1052–1053.
[12] V. Bobek, Anticoagulant and fibrinolytic drugs—possible agents in treatment of lung cancer? Anticancer Agents Med. Chem. 12 (6) (2012) 580–588.
[13] P. Rothwell, F.G. Fowkes, J.F. Belch, H. Ogawa, C.P. Warlow, et al., Effect of daily aspirin on long-term risk of death due to cancer: analysis of individual patient data from randomized trials, Lancet 377 (2011) 31–41.
[14] T. Grint, A.M. Riley, S.J. Mills, B.V.L. Potter, S.T. Safrany, Fibrinogen—A possible extracellular target for inositol phosphates, Messenger 1 (2) (2012) 160–166.
[15] L.R. Zacharski, D.L. Ornstein, Heparin and cancer, Thromb. Haemost. 80 (1) (1998) 10–23.
[16] J.C. Wereldsma, E.D. Bruggink, W.S. Meijer, J.A. Roukema, W.L. van Putten, Adjuvant portal liver infusion in colorectal cancer with 5-fluorouracil/heparin versus urokinase versus control. Results of a prospective randomized clinical trial (colorectal adenocarcinoma trial I), Cancer 65 (3) (1990) 425–432.
[17] D.H. Che, K.Y. Cao, I.H. Shang, Y.C. Man, Y. Yu, The efficacy and safety of low-molecular-weight-heparin use for cancer treatment; a meta-analysis, Eur. J. Intern. Med. 24 (5) (2013) 433–439.

[18] S. Uppal, E. Hernandez, M. Dutta, V. Dandolu, S. Rose, et al., Prolonged postoperative venous thrombo-embolism prophylaxis is cost-effective in advanced ovarian cancer patients, Gynecol. Oncol. 127 (3) (2012) 631–637.

[19] J. Lieb, Antidepressants, prostaglandins and the prevention and treatment of cancer, Med. Hypotheses 69 (3) (2007) 684–689.

[20] D.Y. Lu, T.R. Lu, Antidepressants can be only used as assistant therapy in cancer treatment, Med. Hypotheses 70 (2008) 204–205.

[21] M.H. Teicher, C. Glod, J. O, Emergence of intense suicidal preoccupation during fluoxetine treatment, Am. J. Psychiatry 147 (2) (1990) 207–210.

[22] D.Y. Lu, J. Ding, T.R. Lu, May genetic factors play a role in the risk of antidepressant-induced suicide? Med. Hypotheses 69 (6) (2007) 1380–1381.

[23] D.Y. Lu, T.R. Lu, P.P. Zhu, Undesired neural side-effects of a drug, a chemical and genetic interrelated problem, Central Nervous Syst. Agents Med. Chem. 10 (2) (2010) 108–112.

[24] D.Y. Lu, T.R. Lu, Importance of genomic studies for drug withdrawal with mental toxicities, Drug Ther. Stud. 1 (1) (2011) e11.

[25] D.Y. Lu, T.R. Lu, P.P. Zhu, Genetics in neural toxicities of drugs, Central Nervous Syst. Agents Med. Chem. 12 (4) (2012) 250–253.

[26] The Emperor's Medical Experience. *Questions and Answers* (黄帝内经)。

[27] G. Yang, X. Li, X. Li, L. Wang, J. Li, et al., Traditional Chinese medicine in cancer care: a review of case series published in the Chinese literature, Evid. Based Complement. Altern. Med. 751046 (2012).

[28] E. Manheimer, S. Wieland, E. Kimbrough, K. Cheng, B.M. Berman, Evidence from the cochrane collaboration for traditional chinese medicine therapies, J. Altern. Complement. Med. 15 (9) (2009) 1001–1014.

[29] L.C. Lo, C.Y. Chen, S.T. Chen, H.C. Chen, T.C. Lee, et al., Therapeutic efficacy of traditional Chinese medicine, Shen-Mai San, in cancer patients undergoing chemotherapy or radiotherapy: study protocol for a randomized, double-blind, placebo-controlled trial, Trials 13 (1) (2012) 232.

[30] X.Q. Li, C.Q. Ling, Chinese herbal medicine for side effects of transarterial chemoembolization in liver cancer patients: a systematic review and meta-analysis, Zhong Xi Yi Jie He Xue Bao (J. Chin. Integr. Med.) 10 (12) (2012) 1341–1362.

[31] G. Dennert, M. Horneber, Selenium for alleviating the side effects of chemotherapy, radiotherapy and surgery in cancer patients, Cochrane Database Syst. Rev. 3 (2006) CD005037.

[32] B. Lipinski, Rationale for the treatment of cancer with sodium selenite, Med. Hypotheses 64 (4) (2005) 806–810.

[33] G. Nicolson, Lipid replacement/antioxidant therapy as an adjunct supplement to reduce the adverse effects of cancer therapy and restore mitochondrial function, Pathol. Oncol. Res. 11 (3) (2005) 139–144.

8 Cost-effectiveness considerations

8.1 Background

The running cost of clinical cancer treatment has risen dramatically. It is a huge burden on government budgets and individual cancer patients' expenditure. In the past, we have often created costly and not always very effective new drugs and methodologies and wasted human resources on their development. This greatly increases therapeutic costs. Now some countries, such as USA or Japan, are overburdened with the high expense of medical resources in human diagnosis and therapy, especially for human cancer therapy. Thus, we ought to carefully check our spending in line with positive treatment outcomes. The term 'cost-effective strategy' has been denominated and systematically studied. The costs of anticancer drug developments and licensing are skyrocketing, approximate 1-1.8 billions USD in US [1,2]. So the anticancer drug costs in hospitals are also very expensive. Cost-effective study cancer therapy is an indispensable part of cancer therapy, especially for ICC.

Cost-effectiveness is a long-standing medical problem, pervasive in all areas of disease control and there is also an early concern about the mathematics of cost-effective evaluations of diagnosis and drug responses in ICC. Increasing efforts to develop ICC are generally shadowed by rising diagnostic and drug-response prediction costs, and the expense of anticancer drugs. Systematic evaluation of the relationship between the running costs and benefits of ICC is crucial for updating ICC systems and making ICC available in the long run. Since the cost of anticancer and antimetastatic therapy is a critical matter, the balance between cost and effectiveness is an unavoidable ICC research project [3–9].

8.2 Routine cost of cancer chemotherapy

8.2.1 Background

Routine cancer chemotherapy is expensive. Generally the cost of a course of cancer therapy is more than 10,000 USD. If a patient needs antibody therapy, let alone ICC strategies, the running cost of cancer chemotherapy will exceed 10,000 USD. So the study of cost-effectiveness is an important task, both to save cancer patients' money and to optimize the therapy.

8.3 Calculation of cost-effectiveness

The cost-effectiveness ratio is calculated as the ratio of costs to quality-adjusted life-years (QALYs). An incremental cost-effectiveness ratio (ICER) of <₡20,000 is regarded as cost-effective in developed countries [4]. The ICER might be much lower

Personalized Cancer Chemotherapy.

for cost-effectiveness in developing countries. Apart from cost, the toxicities of a therapy must also be examined when selecting a therapy. Some drugs, such as antibodies, are very expensive, and render the calculated ICER higher than an ICER of chemical drugs only. It seems as if chemical drugs are better than antibodies. However, the overall survival rate using antibodies plus chemical drugs is much longer than the overall survival rate using chemical drugs alone. The financial conditions of cancer patients must decide what kind of a therapy a patient may choose [5].

In view of the $10,000-plus expenditure on common cycles of drug combination and hospital residence fees, the cancer biomarker or bioinformatics detection fee ($100-5,000) is relatively cost-effective. After detecting cancer biomarkers, it will increase the quality-adjusted life-year (QALY) of cancer patients, especially in some early-stage cancers [6,7].

For late-stage cancer patients, antimetastatic drugs, targeting formed metastatic foci, should be used. In antimetastatic drug development there is currently a worldwide lack of licensed drugs. This type of drug research, development and clinical utilization must be boosted [10–13].

8.3.1 Cost-effectiveness study from consideration of methodology of individualized cancer chemotherapy

A cost-effectiveness study, from consideration of the methodology of individualized cancer chemotherapy is a basic aspect of individualized cancer chemotherapy. There are many different options from different methodologies of individualized cancer chemotherapy. Which is the best methodology for a specific patient? One consideration is the clinical situation of a patient, and the other consideration is cost.

8.3.2 Cost-effectiveness of different predictive methodologies

In the genotyping of different polymorphisms of genes of a metabolizing enzyme or of drug response molecules, which one might be more suitable for a patient and how much single nucleotide polymorphism (SNP) should we detect that can make costs balance and assure beneficial outcomes. This is a new subject. There are many SNPs in a specific gene, some are important to therapy, some are often negligible for drug-response prediction. In clinical practice, how to genotype these genes of metabolizing enzymes and drug targeting molecules is also a problem of cost-effectiveness. Relevant information and experience are based on previous experimental data and accumulation of clinical evidence [14]. If there is enough clinical evidence of polymorphism of some genes responsible for some varied drug responses, the doctor then may decide to perform genotyping of these genes in routine ICC strategies.

For drug sensitivity testing, the running cost of *in vivo* drug sensitivity test methodology is several-fold higher than that of *in vitro* drug sensitivity test methodology. So *in vivo* drug sensitivity test methodology ought to be used less frequently.

The evaluation of the cost-effectiveness of individualized cancer chemotherapy can be different according to different systems. The evaluation of the effects of individualized cancer chemotherapy covers both inhibition of primary tumors and survival benefits. For drug sensitivity tests, it is often reported that there is a marked benefit in regard to the inhibition of primary tumors but that, however, there are no survival benefits from this method, even though the primary tumor is inhibited [15]. The calculation of the cost-effectiveness of drug sensitivity tests will vary according to different evaluation systems.

On the other hand, treatment effects to primary tumors may differ from treatment effects to metastatic tumors with the use of different drug categories. The intimate relationship of these two must be carefully analyzed according to patients' clinical situations and the anticancer or antimetastatic drugs being used.

The calculation of cost-effectiveness, based as it is on clinical data and used to predict therapeutic benefits, will improve, develop and be more useful as time goes by.

8.4 The keys to the study of cost-effectiveness in individualized cancer chemotherapy

Calculation of cost-effectiveness in individualized cancer chemotherapy is no easy task. The cost and benefits of each category of diagnosis and anticancer therapy must be precisely known. This is a system for designing a therapeutic regime based on the consideration of budget and of patients' clinical situations. Drug sensitivity testing, or genotyping of drug response molecules, or metabolizing enzyme genes calls for a certain amount of money. However, their survival benefits are conditional and not consistent. Some gene polymorphism—another point—is absent in some ethnic groups—ethnic frequency equals zero (Table 8.1), so in these ethnic groups, there is no need to genotype these gene polymorphisms before initiating therapy [14]. So the genotyping of drug response molecules or metabolizing enzyme genes needs different pharmacogenetics protocols according to patients' ethnic groups and running costs. Economic and ethnic consideration of patients' real situations are essential. In the

Table 8.1 **Ethnic frequency (%) of allelic variants in CYP2B6**

Allelic variants	SNP	Caucasian	African American	Asian	Hispanic
CYP2B6*2	C64T	5.3–9.0	0	4.7	
CYP2B6*3	C777A	0.5		0	
CYP2B6*4	A785G	4.0–32.6	16.7	9.3	14.3
CYP2B6*5	C1459T	9.5–13	9.0	1.1	0
CYP2B6*6	G516T A785G	25.6		16.4	
CYP2B6*7	G516T A785G C1459T	0–0.3		0	
CYP2B6*8	A415G	1.0	0	0	0

SNY, single nucleotide polymorphism Ref 12.

past, anticoagulant prophylaxis in operative ovarian cancer patients has been proved cost-effective (chapter 7).

Amongst different categories of expenditure in individualized cancer chemotherapy, the choice of an excellent drug is the first step. Methodologies such as drug sensitivity test, biomarker detecting or pharmacogenomics are further steps that may perfect a therapy, but will also increase the cost. Whether a therapy can be beneficial always depends on cost and patients' clinical situations. If a cancer patient is old (over 65 years of age) and in a late stage, use only of antimetastatic drugs and anticoagulant or traditional Chinese medicine assistant therapy seems more acceptable. If a patient is young (15–35 years old) or in early stages, the success of a therapy is more likely and 100% ICC seems the best way.

8.5 Future trends

The consideration of cost-effectiveness for drug combinations or assistant therapy is one aspect of a clinician's work and of basic cancer chemotherapy studies, especially when costly drugs are to be used.

In the future, software will be perfected which may help in making satisfactory decisions on optimized therapeutic outcomes before individualized cancer chemotherapy begins. Standard software must be constantly improved and updated, based on essential data.

8.6 Conclusion

The ultimate goal of the study of cost-effectiveness in individualized cancer chemotherapy is to maximize therapeutic outcomes at minimum cost. The cost of prediction of drug responses in individualized cancer chemotherapy (100-5,000 USD) is lower than the cost of some expensive anticancer or antimetastatic drugs and hospital residence. Overall, individualized cancer chemotherapy is generally cost-effective, especially for young and early-stage cancer patients. The more appropriate the use of funds and prediction of anticancer drug responses, the more therapeutic the benefits that may be achieved for a specific cancer patient.

References

[1] S.C. Gupta, B. Sung, S. Prasad, B.B. Aggarwal, Cancer drug discovery by repurposing: teaching new tricks to old dogs, Trends Pharmacol. Sci. 34 (9) (2013) 507–517.

[2] B.A. Ruggeri, F. Camp, S. Miknyoczki, Animal models of disease: Preclinical animal models of cancer and their applications and utility in drug discovery, Biochem. Pharmacol. 87 (2014) 150–161.

[3] D.Y. Lu, X.L. Chen, J. Ding, Individualized cancer chemotherapy integrating drug sensitivity tests, pathological profile analysis and computational coordination-an effective strategy to improve clinical treatment, Med. Hypotheses 66 (1) (2006) 45–51.
[4] J.P. Greving, F. Vernooij, S.P.M. Heinz, Y. van der Graaf, E. Buskens, Is centralization of ovarian cancer care warranted? A cost-effectiveness analysis, Gynecol. Oncol. 113 (1) (2009) 68–74.
[5] J.L. Lesnock, C. Farris, T.C. Krivak, K.J. Smith, M. Markman, Consolidation paclitaxel is more cost-effective than bevacizumab following upfront treatment of advanced epithelial ovarian cancer, Gynecol. Oncol. 122 (3) (2011) 473–478.
[6] V.P. Retèl, M.A. Joore, M. Knauer, S.C. Linn, M. Hauptmann, et al., Cost-effectiveness of the 70-gene signature versus St. Gallen guidelines and Adjuvant Online for early breast cancer, Eur. J. Cancer 46 (8) (2010) 1382–1391.
[7] A. Naeim, E.B. Keeler, Is adjuvant therapy for older patients with node (-) early breast cancer cost-effective? Crit. Rev. Oncol. Hematol. 53 (1) (2005) 81–89.
[8] S. Uppal, E. Hernandez, M. Dutta, V. Dandolu, S. Rose, et al., Prolonged postoperative venous thrombo-embolism prophylaxis is cost-effective in advanced ovarian cancer patients, Gynecol. Oncol. 127 (3) (2012) 631–637.
[9] T.S. Foster, J.D. Miller, M.K. Boye, M.B. Blieden, R. Gidwani, et al., The economic burden of metastatic breast cancer: a systematic review of literature from developed countries, Cancer Treat. Rev. 37 (6) (2011) 405–415.
[10] S. Valastyan, R.A. Weinberg, Tumor metastasis: molecular insights and evolving paradigms, Cell 147 (2) (2011) 275–292.
[11] D.Y. Lu, T.R. Lu, S. Cao, Cancer metastases and clinical therapies, Cell. Dev. Biol. 1 (4) (2012) e110.
[12] D.Y. Lu, T.R. Lu, H.Y. Wu, New Insights into individualized antimetastatic therapy, Adv. Tech. Biol. Med. 1 (1) (2013) 106.
[13] D.Y. Lu, T.R. Lu, H.Y. Wu, S. Cao, Cancer metastases treatments, Curr. Drug Ther. 8 (1) (2013) 24–29.
[14] J.F. Deeken, W.D. Figg, S.E. Bates, A. Sparreboom, Toward individualized treatment: prediction of anticancer drug disposition and toxicity with pharmacogenetics, Anticancer Drugs 18 (2) (2007) 111–126.
[15] D.Y. Lu, T.R. Lu, X.L. Chen, J. Ding, Individualized cancer chemotherapy, in: M.M. Shoja, P.S. Agutter, R.S. Tubbs, M. Ghanei, K. Ghabili et al. (Eds.), Hypotheses in Clinical Medicine, Nova Science Publishers, Hauppage, NY, 2012, pp. 199–216. Chapter 13.

Discussion

9

Different individualized cancer chemotherapy (ICC) strategies are employed in clinical cancer treatments. We must therefore understand the pros and cons of each individualized cancer chemotherapy strategy from different angles so as to make good judgments and predictions of drug responses and clinical outcomes. In this chapter, we will discuss each of the ICC systems, especially the pitfalls readers may face.

9.1 Drug sensitivity testing

Drug sensitivity was at the core of individualized cancer chemotherapy in the past. Before the advent of drug sensitivity testing, cancer clinicians made therapeutic decisions on an empirical basis in terms of the pathological features of the cancer, rather than by thorough understanding and evaluation of individual tumor and human responses to anticancer drugs in clinics. Since the introduction of drug sensitivity testing, cancer clinicians have become more important in cancer treatment. Several points have been made:

1. When tumors acquire MDR and become refractory or recurrent after first-line chemotherapy, a poor clinical prognosis seems inevitable. Drug sensitivity testing seems to be useful for these cancer patients [1–2].
2. The utility of drug sensitivity testing can be shown by another scenario. It is said that there is a marginal benefit in terms of overall survival for colon cancer patients with normal prognoses, but that there are marked survival benefits for colon cancer patients with poor prognoses, especially those with tumors over-expressing HER2 [3]. In such a scenario, drug sensitivity testing is optimal for both drug responses to primary tumors and to calculate survival benefits in cancer patients with no formed metastatic foci, and is best suited for the latter.

Many studies show the favorable or beneficial effects of employing drug sensitivity tests in clinics. The drug response rates of patients are improved in approximately 10-50% of cancer patients, but survival benefits are reported to be relatively small [2,4–5]. This is the main reason why the effectiveness of drug sensitivity testing is contentious.

There are two main causes of this phenomenon:

1. There is a possibility of a tumor acquiring MDA quickly. Thus a patient's tumor will regrow very quickly.
2. Cancer patients die of tumor metastases, while drug sensitivity testing tests drug responses mostly to primary tumors. So there is no improvement in patients' survival rates.

Although drug sensitivity tests have not been routinely used in clinics, the debates about them continue and reports on their benefits vary from patient to patient. We should remain optimistic about their further development and utility.

Personalized Cancer Chemotherapy.

More clinicians should be encouraged and trained to use the drug-sensitivity-testing strategy. With such an approach, along with perfection of methodologies, the strategy will be transferred from bench to bedside. Several important considerations in developing drug-sensitivity-testing strategies will need to be taken into account:

9.1.1 Technical considerations for improvement [2]

1. The number of drugs available for choosing:
   Increasing the number of drugs available for choice on the basis of a single drug sensitivity test will help in selecting the drugs best suited for chemotherapy [1].
   Drug sensitivity tests are more suitable for selection of cytotoxic anticancer drugs.
2. The simplification of drug sensitivity tests:
   We propose that drug sensitivity tests be simplified [1]. Ulukaya [6] challenges this view by arguing that simplification of the drug –sensitivity-test protocol would lead to poor test performance. However, there may be no relationship between therapeutic outcome and simplicity of protocol. We argue here again that with a deeper understanding of the nature of cancer cells after systematic scientific investigations, we can utilize more appropriate and simpler conditions for growing and testing tumor cells. In ordinary hospitals, it is impractical to support very sophisticated protocols. The shortening and simplification of drug-sensitivity tests without compromising their effects must be a future trend. The simpler the drug-sensitivity-test protocol, the more hospitals can implement drug sensitivity testing [2].
3. Selection of clonal or stem cells in drug sensitivity tests

The success or failure of a chemotherapy regime is determined by a number of clonal or stem cells in a tumor tissue [7–8]. Thus drug sensitivity tests aiming at determining drug response against clonal or stem cancer cells might be more useful and suitable for hospital drug sensitivity testing routine in future. A new stage of *in vitro* drug sensitivity testing should be introduced, focusing on these tumor types for predicting drug response to a tumor tissue.

Many technical details of drug sensitivity testing will determine the fate of individualized cancer chemotherapy. These technical details must be carefully observed and every detail of drug sensitivity tests adhered to.

9.2 The development of cancer biomarker detection

Whether there is a relationship between cancer biomarker levels in individual tumor specimens and drug response outcomes among cancer patients is difficult to define. The central point in this issue is to identify the original or causative cancer biomarkers in a specific tumor tissue.

There are two important approaches to genetic, molecular and bioinformatics-based ICC strategies. The first one is to detect as many polymorphisms or cytological levels of biomarkers as possible at the least possible cost. The second is to pinpoint the original or causative biomarkers as clearly as possible by mathematical, genetic or biological means. The more successfully we can pinpoint these original genes or molecules, the more appropriate anticancer and antimetastatic drugs we can correctly choose and the better we can predict anticancer drug responses, especially for monotherapy or ribonucleic acid interference (RNAi) agents. These two approaches need to be systemized or optimized, e.g. standard chips and techniques [2,9] and genetic analysis software are waiting to be developed and perfected. Finally, the following priorities for improving ICC strategy are suggested and emphasized:

1. to sketch routine ICC procedures in a formed diagram;
2. to develop novel applicable equations and calculating systems;
3. to design automatic protocols to save labor that can be universally usable in conventional hospitals [2].

Genetic, molecular or bioinformatics detection of human cancer biomarkers for predicting drug responses are modern concepts and will develop quickly in future.

The results of a recent genomic study of >3,000 tumors across 26 cancer types show that only 1/4 of these tumors contain known cancer genes [10]. This means that most tumors are caused by undefined cancer genes. Thus, there is great potential for further investigations of cancer biomarkers.

9.3 Pharmacogenetics or pharmacogenomics

Pharmacogenetics or pharmacogenomics modalities in clinics can be used to tell how to use a specific anticancer drug, but pharmacogenetics or pharmacogenomics is not useful for telling why this anticancer drug must be used in a specific tumor origin. It is drug sensitivity testing or cancer biomarker detecting that can tell which drugs must be used in a specific tumor origin. Pharmacogenetics or pharmacogenomics methods give only information of possible drug response genes or molecules for a defined anticancer drug in a cancer patient.

9.4 Antimetastatic therapy

Cancer patients' deaths are commonly decided by cancer metastasis. So individualized antimetastatic therapies might usefully be a future trend.

We have emphasized two strategies of individualized antimetastatic therapies:

1. individualized antimetastatic therapies in response to metastatic cascade [11–12];
2. special drugs targeting formed metastasis [13–14].

We propose that cancer patients' survival rates can be improved by applying these two strategies.

9.5 Should antimetastatic drugs be offered to all cancer patients?

Cancer metastases do not occur in all patients. 60% of patients suffer from those tumor types with low metastatic rates [15]. These patients will have good survival expectancy and do not require additional antimetastatic therapy. Surgery or therapy targeting primary tumors will suffice. However, in some other cases (30–40% of cancer patients), it is not known if a specific individual will metastasize or not. In some cases, metastasized tumors have been found when patients are diagnosed with cancer. Here, there are two main options:

1. find out whether there are some metastatic gene signatures in primary tumors [16–18];
2. treat metastatic foci with more active drugs. This is the central problem, and will be discussed in the following sections.

9.6 Drug combinations

Mounting experimental data and clinical evidence suggest it might be optimal to use drug combinations in controlling tumor growth and metastasis. However, the toxicities of drug combinations to humans are increased alongside the increase in drug numbers. Drug sensitivity tests, cancer biomarker detection and pharmacogenetics are designed to select effective drugs from anticancer drug arsenals and to discard ineffective drugs. They can establish a good balance between drug activity and toxicity.

Each anticancer drug has its own effects and toxicities [19]. It is not always the truth that more drugs are better than a single drug. Single drug or drug combination options must be carefully assessed and judged, based on established medical theory, individualized cancer chemotherapy strategies and the clinical situations of cancer patients.

9.7 Assistant therapies

There are many success stories of cancer patients' survival rates being increased by assistant therapies. Most assistant therapies in ICC are cost-effectiven and also effective for late-stage cancer patients. However, assistant therapies must work with traditional cancer therapies, or their anticancer effect will be reduced or nullified.

9.8 Overall considerations

Most anticancer drugs can be divided into two categories: cytotoxic and cytostatic [20]. To predict the possible effects of cytotoxic anticancer drugs on cancer tissues, the best method is drug sensitivity testing or pharmacogenomics. To predict the possible effects of cytostatic agents or biotherapy, it is better to detect cancer biomarkers or cancer bioinformatics. Cancer biomarkers and bioinformatics can reveal which cancer pathways might be targeted.

Many strategies for individualized cancer chemotherapies are complementary with one another. Clinically, we can apply two or three types of ICC strategy in one cancer patient. Cancer patients must be treated according to their clinical situation and financial condition. The more familiar we are with all aspects of individualized cancer chemotherapy strategies, the better we can help and successfully treat cancer patients. However, these therapies must be based on cost-effectiveness evaluations.

Since we cannot possibly use all of these strategies for one patient, amongst the different types of ICC, which ICC strategy is the best? Each of them has its own advantages and disadvantages. At present no one type of ICC strategy is obviously advantageous over the others. Also, no available ICC strategy has been good enough to significantly increase the patient's survival compared with conventional therapy. So we desperately need some magic moves to improve present ICC strategies or create new types to integrate the advantages of all ICC types. Great efforts have been made towards fulfillment of ICC, but many substantial obstacles still need to be surmounted. The chief problem preventing this fulfillment at the moment is that on many occasions there is almost no improvement in survival rates in late-stage cancer patients, in spite of applications of ICC. Still, this can be a future miracle if we can overcome this and perfect a successful ICC. Are we ready? [21]

References

[1] D.Y. Lu, X.L. Chen, J. Ding, Individualized cancer chemotherapy integrating drug sensitivity tests, pathological profile analysis and computational coordination-an effective strategy to improve clinical treatment, Med. Hypotheses 66 (1) (2006) 45–51.

[2] D.Y. Lu, T.R. Lu, X.L. Chen, J. Ding, Individualized cancer chemotherapy, in: M.M. Shoja, P.S. Agutter, R.S. Tubbs, M. Ghanei, K. Ghabili et al. (Eds.), Hypotheses in Clinical Medicine, Nova Science Publisher, Hauppage, NY, 2012, pp. 199–216. chapter 13.

[3] R. Kim, M. Emi, K. Tanabe, Y. Uchida, T. Toge, Chemosensitivity testing for gastrointestinal cancer: survival benefit potential and limitations, Anticancer Drugs 14 (9) (2003) 715–723.

[4] D.D. Von Hoff, J.F. Sandbach, G.M. Clark, J.N. Turner, B.F. Forseth, et al., Selection of cancer chemotherapy for a patient by an in vitro assay versus a clinician, J. Natl. Cancer. Inst. 82 (2) (1990) 110–116.

[5] P. Venesmaa, O. Ylikorkala, Subrenal capsule assay in selection of chemotherapy after operation for recurrent ovarian cancer, Br. J. Cancer 63 (1) (1991) 84–86.

[6] S. Ugurel, D. Schadendorf, C. Pföhler, K. Neuber, A. Thoelke, et al., In vitro drug sensitivity predicts response and survival after individualized sensitivity-directed chemotherapy in metastatic melanoma: a multicenter phase II trial of the Dermatologic Cooperative Oncology Group, Clin. Cancer Res. 12 (18) (2006) 5454–5463.

[7] J.S. Yakisich, Challenges and limitations of targeting cancer stem cells and/or the tumour microenvironment, Drugs Ther. Stud. 2 (1) (2012) e10.

[8] Y. Takamura, et al., Prediction of chemotherapeutic response by collagen gel droplet embedded culture-drug sensitivity test in human breast cancers, Int. J. Cancer 98 (3) (2002) 450–455.

[9] V.P. Retèl, M. A. Joore, M. Knauer, S.C. Linn, M. Hauptmann, et al., Cost-effectiveness of the 70-gene signature versus St. Gallen guidelines and adjuvant online for early breast cancer, Eur. J. Cancer 46 (8) (2010) 1382–1391.

[10] E.S. Lander, Initial impact of the sequencing of the human genome, Nature 470 (2011) 187–197.

[11] D.Y. Lu, F.G. Wu, Z.M. Shen, T.R. Lu, H.Y. Wu, et al., Different spontaneous pulmonary metastasis inhibitions against lewis lung carcinoma in mice by bisdioxopiperazine compounds of different treatment schedules, Scientia Pharm. 78 (2010) 13–20.

[12] D.Y. Lu, Y.C. Xi, Antimetastatic therapies according to metastatic cascade, Adv. Pharm. Drug Safety 1 (2012) e107.

[13] D.Y. Lu, T.R. Lu, S. Cao, Cancer metastases and clinical therapies, Cell. Dev. Biol. 1 (4) (2012) e110.

[14] D.Y. Lu, T.R. Lu, H.Y. Wu, S. Cao, Cancer metastases treatments, Curr. Drug Ther. 8 (1) (2013) 24–29.

[15] R. Siegel, E. Ward, O. Brawley, A. Jamal, Cancer statistics 2011, CA Cancer J. Clin. 61 (2011) 212–236.

[16] G. Finak, N. Bertos, F. Pepin, S. Sadekova, M. Souleimanova, et al., Stromal gene expression predicts clinical outcome in breast cancer, Nat. Med. 14 (5) (2008) 518–527.

[17] W. Wang, S. Goswami, K. Lapidus, A.L. Wells, J.B. Wyckoff, et al., Identification and testing of a gene expression signature of invasive carcinoma cells within primary mammary tumors, Cancer Res. 64 (2004) 8585–8594.

[18] D.Y. Lu, T.R. Lu, S. Cao, Individualized cancer chemotherapy by detecting cancer biomarkers, Metabolomics 2 (5) (2012) e121.

[19] D.Y. Lu, T.R. Lu, J. Ding, Employing new mathematical models and equations to evaluate risk-benefit criteria of clinical therapeutics, Online J. Bio. Sci. 7 (1) (2007) 1–2.

[20] A.W. Millar, K.P. Lynch, Rethinking clinical trials for cytostatic drugs, Nat. Rev. Cancer 3 (7) (2003) 540–545.

[21] D.Y. Lu, T.R. Lu, X.L. Chen, Individualized cancer chemotherapy, are we ready for that yet? Metabolomics 2 (2012) e113.

Conclusion

10

Most ICC strategies are imperfect now and in their emerging stages, owing to unsatisfactory clinical outcomes and higher costs than those of conventional chemotherapies. There are several key factors behind these unsatisfactory results. This book gives a panorama of currently applied ICC strategies and homes in on the drawbacks of every strategy. It serves as a platform for discussion and promotion of these ICC strategies in future.

Drug sensitivity testing and pharmacogenomics are the mainstream of current individualized cancer chemotherapy (ICC) [1]. By analyzing different available ICC strategies, we suggest the equal importance of every type of ICC strategy.

However, drug sensitivity testing is unsatisfactory now. Survival rates have improved very little in late-stage cancer patients, in spite of the utilization of drug-sensitivity testing. Many factors, such as increasing drug numbers in drug-sensitivity testing, the development of more active and specific anticancer or antimetastatic drugs, may ameliorate this [1–2]. The more effective and selective anticancer or antimetastatic drugs are developed, the more favorable outcomes different ICC strategies may offer, because there are better choices of drug armaments.

Sequencing cancer genomes has gradually increased our power to pinpoint tumor biomarkers. Detection of alterations of tumor genetics, transcripts, protein, glycoprotein or other types of cancer molecules in clinical tumor samples will need less and less money and more bioinformation in future. For instance, the speed of drafting genomes has increased 15,000-50,000 times compared with the first successful drafting of the human genome 10 years ago [3–5]. Cancer biomarker or bioinformatics detection-based ICC strategy will also change with the times and will cost less with technical innovations, making it potentially one of the most valuable ICC strategies in the future.

A recent genomic study of >3,000 tumors across 26 cancer types showed that only 1/4 of these tumors contain known cancer genes [5] and therefore most tumors are caused by undefined cancer genes. There is therefore great potential for further investigations of cancer biomarkers.

Pharmacogenomics nowadays is like a luxury item. It can be purchased or neglected, depending on patients' financial conditions, or the drugs being used. Pharmacogenomics, commonly named personalized medicine, is currently regarded as the most important source of individualized cancer chemotherapy. Though we can foresee about how active a drug can be in a human body, we cannot know if this drug is the most appropriate for a specific tumor tissue. To put it another way, anticancer drugs are multi-gene-targeted. We can analyze one drug in one gene polymorphism, but we cannot know this drug's action on other gene functions or polymorphisms. This is one of the biggest drawbacks in this area [6]. For the success of pharmacogenetics and pharmacogenomics, first enough experimental or clinical data must be accumulated and a solid relationship built between genes and drug responses to tumor tissue. Our present knowledge of genetic influences on drug responses and toxicity are no more than one fifth of what we ought to know. We may in time obtain enough genotype-phenotype association or genetic-drug responses relationship information to serve the goal of increasing cancer patients' survival by means of clinical pharmacogenetic applications.

Now individualized cancer chemotherapy (ICC) can be mainly divided into drug sensitivity testing, pharmacogenomics and cancer biomarker detection (Figure 10.1). In future, new disciplines, such as individualized antimetastatic chemotherapy and individualized assistant chemotherapy, may come into being. ICC has been evolving from drug sensitivity testing into a multi-disciplinary, more sophisticated enterprise. However, it is still in its infant stage. It must in time be implemented into knowledge-based systematic structures. This book is only a medium to help readers understand the core of cancer treatment and to invite new light on this matter.

The other huge drawback of current individualized cancer chemotherapy is the design of anticancer drugs against primary tumors rather than against metastatic lesions. Individualized antimetastatic chemotherapy may be the key to the future strategy of ICC. From the clinical point of view, 90% of cancer patients die of metastases. So this pathological feature, of cancer metastasis, is more powerfully linked with patients' survival and its treatment must be boosted in future individualized antimetastatic chemotherapies [7–10]. This type of ICC is especially important.

In order to understand all ICC strategies in depth, we urgently need well-designed, prospective, double-blind studies to systematically evaluate all possibilities and advance this strategy in a race against time.

The study of cost-effective drug combination and biotherapy is a core aspect of individualized cancer chemotherapy. In future, we must use low-cost, highly effective anticancer drugs in individualized cancer chemotherapy. Considering the more-than-$10,000 expenditure on common cycles of drug combination, the biomarker detection fee ($100-5,000) is relatively cost-effective. After detecting cancer biomarkers, it will increase the quality-adjusted life-year (QALY) of cancer patients, especially in some early-stage cancer [10–11]. Almost each of the presently used ICC strategies is cost-effective today compared with conventional cancer chemotherapy.

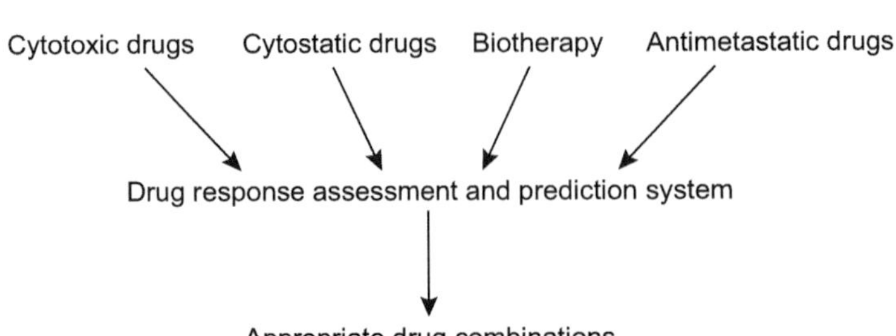

Figure 10.1 General scheme of individualized cancer chemotherapy.

From the perspective of the current situation of ICC strategy utilization, this utilization has only a less-than-15% rate of occurrence. A lot of hospitals never try any ICC strategies. In future, ICC strategies should be improved and perfected for survival rate benefit, or even cure, of late-stage cancer patients. The more we try ICC strategies in clinics, the more satisfactory outcomes we may obtain. More cancer clinicians should notice and apply these strategies, because ICC strategies are the best way to treat and cure cancer patients.

The ultimate goal of ICC strategies is to markedly decrease cancer deaths. ICC strategies seem to be one of the best options for cancer treatment. No matter which type of ICC strategy is used in clinics, it ought to be effective and in a reasonable cost range. Following this rule, other better new ICC strategies may be innovated and better organized. In the past 10 years, the focus of ICC strategies has shifted from drug-sensitivity testing only into pharmacogenomics. In the next decade, we hypothesize that ICC strategies will be transformed from anticancer drug pharmacogenomics into cancer biomarker-oriented therapy or individualized antimetastatic therapy.

ICC strategies are a good way to treat cancer patients and will become routine in hospitals. But so far, no available ICC strategy has been sufficiently effective to significantly increase patients' survival rates compared with conventional therapy. We need some 'magic moves' to create avant-garde techniques to improve present ICC strategies or to create state-of-the-art types of ICC strategies that integrate the advantages of all ICC types. Although great efforts have been made in fulfillment of ICC, many major obstacles remain. There is little improvement in cancer patients' survival rates, in spite of the application of some types of ICC. If we perfect ICC strategies, we can anticipate what will seem miraculous [12].

References

[1] D.Y. Lu, T. R. Lu, X. L. Chen, J. Ding, et al., Individualized cancer chemotherapy, in: M.M. Shoja, P.S. Agutter, R.S. Tubbs, M. Ghanei, K. Ghabili, et al., (Eds.), Hypotheses in Clinical Medicine, Nova Science Publisher, Hauppage, NY, 2012, pp. 199–216. chapter 13.

[2] D.Y. Lu, X. L. Chen, J. Ding, Individualized cancer chemotherapy integrating drug sensitivity tests, pathological profile analysis and computational coordination-an effective strategy to improve clinical treatment, Med. Hypotheses 66 (1) (2006) 45–51.

[3] F. Collins, Has the revolution arrived? Nature 464 (2010) 674–675.

[4] J.C. Venter, Multiple personal genomes await, Nature 464 (2010) 676–677.

[5] E.S. Lander, Initial impact of the sequencing of the human genome, Nature 470 (2011) 187–197.

[6] R.S. Huang, M. J. Ratain, Pharmacogenetics and pharmacogenomics of anticancer drugs, CA: A Cancer J. Clin. 59 (2009) 42–55.

[7] D.Y. Lu, T. R. Lu, S. Cao, Cancer metastases and clinical therapies, Cell. Dev. Biol. 1 (4) (2012) e110.

[8] S. Valastyan, R. A. Weinberg, Tumor metastasis: molecular insights and evolving paradigms, Cell 147 (2) (2011) 275–292.

[9] D.Y. Lu, T. R. Lu, H. Y. Wu, S. Cao, Cancer metastasis treatments, Curr. Drug Ther. 8 (1) (2013) 24–29.

[10] V.P. Retèl, M. A. Joore, M. Knauer, S. C. Linn, M. Hauptmann, et al., Cost-effectiveness of the 70-gene signature versus St. Gallen guidelines and adjuvant online for early breast cancer, Eur. J. Cancer 46 (8) (2010) 1382–1391.

[11] A. Naeim, E. B. Keeler, Is adjuvant therapy for older patients with node (-) early breast cancer cost-effective? Crit. Rev. Oncol. Hematol. 53 (1) (2005) 81–89.

[12] D.Y. Lu, T. R. Lu, X. L. Chen, Individualized cancer chemotherapy, are we ready for that yet? Metabolomics 2 (2012) e113.

FSC
www.fsc.org
MIX
Papier | Fördert gute Waldnutzung
FSC® C083411

Kolibri 360 GmbH
Ferdinand-Jühlke-Straße 7
99095 Erfurt, Deutschland
produktsicherheit@kolibri360.de